Sassy Gal's
How to Lose the Last
Damn
10 Pounds
or 15, 20, 25 . . .

Be Sassy!

Sharon Hulbert

Sassy Gal's
How to Lose the Last *Damn* 10 Pounds
or 15, 20, 25...

How I told all diet gurus, fitness experts, and skinny people to go to hell. Then I killed them, ate them, and still lost weight. You can too!

Sharon Helbert

ALEGCRIS PRESS
Boston, Massachusetts

Published and distributed by
  Alegcris Press, LLC
  P.O. Box 610099
  Newton Highlands, MA 02461

Cover design by David Aldrich
Illustration by Kath Walker
Editing by Erin Brenner
Proofreading by Joanna Eng
Book production by Glenna Collett

This publication contains the opinions and ideas of its author. It is sold with the understanding that the author and publisher are not engaged in rendering health services in the book. The reader should consult his or her own medical and health providers as appropriate before adopting any of the suggestions in this book or drawing inferences from it.

The author and publisher specifically disclaim all responsibility for any liability, loss or risk, personal or otherwise, which is incurred as a consequence, directly or indi-rectly, of the use and application of any of the contents of this book.

Printed in USA

Library of Congress Control Number   2011910968

ISBN-13: 978-0-9836752-6-6

10 9 8 7 6 5 4 3 2 1

Visit us on the web!
  www.sassy-gal.com
  www.alegcrispress.com

This book is dedicated to my family, who made this book possible:

My parents, Clint and Audrey Riegle, who offered loving support and who taught me about spending precious time together, going on adventures and enjoying the outdoors. May we spend many more years together around the campfire.

My husband Russ, who gave me technical expertise and a daily dose of laughter. I am grateful that we share the love of our precious daughters and sweet, gentle collies.

My darling daughters, Alexandra and Christina, who gave me creative inspiration and fostered a "Go-for-it!" attitude. How fortunate I am to be your mom.

Our beloved collies, George and Ginger, who have taught me another dimension to the meaning of love and have been the best walking buddies ever.

I appreciate all of your generous encouragement throughout this journey. Along the way we laughed, became a little sassy, and ultimately learned that the key to our happiness includes a daily piece of chocolate. I am grateful to you for already giving me a lifetime of love.

Contents

Recipes

Coming soon . . .

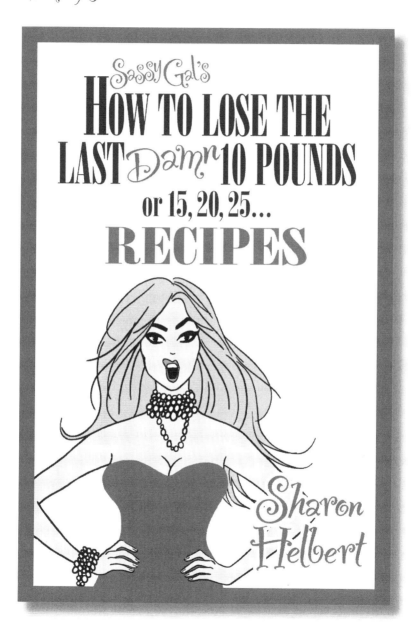

Sassy Gal's
HOW TO LOSE THE LAST Damn 10 POUNDS
or 15, 20, 25...
RECIPES

Sharon
Helbert

Acknowledgments

I would like to thank all the individuals who have contributed so generously towards helping me turn my personal journey into a book that I hope inspires others to change their attitudes about what a healthy lifestyle means to them.

To my Mom, Audrey Riegle—Your endless encouragement and truthfulness while working on this book were so important to me and I thank you. You believed in me, and as your daughter it doesn't get any better than that.

To Erin Brenner—Your skills as an editor provided me with invaluable suggestions and guidance, helping me transform my personal story into a book I'm proud of. Thank you for helping me find my *Sassy* voice, yet also letting me maintain a humorous tone to my writing.

To Glenna Collett—Your savvy business sense and quick decision making guided me through the complex book production process. You are also a pleasure to work with.

To David Aldrich—Your talent for creating beautiful and striking book covers inspired me to choose you. Thank you for designing this incredible "eye-catching" book cover.

To Kath Walker—Your illustrations are so original and creative that I knew immediately that you could help me capture the essence of *Sassy Gal*. Thank you for this fantastic design.

To Joanna Eng—Your skill as proofreader was invaluable. Thank you for joining our team and looking after every detail in such a professional manner.

To Laura Boyer—Your wisdom, combined with your keen sense of humor, was so important to me. You gave me immense confidence for which I am grateful. I also thank you for the precious time we spent together with our families, especially with our daughters.

To my girlfriends—Thank you for being on this lifelong journey with me, and for encouraging me to write my story because you felt I had something to say. Let's go celebrate by enjoying some delicious chocolate cake!

A Few Words . . .

Why I Wrote This Book

I wrote this book because I had a happy ending. I did lose those last damn 10 pounds—without the help of diet gurus, fitness experts, diet pills, weight-loss centers, prepackaged diet foods, spiritual advisors, hypnosis, or duct tape.

I am happier, calmer, and a much kinder person to be around. After all these years, I finally succeeded, and I would like to share my story with you, so you too can have a happy ending.

My Credentials

I am no expert. Nor am I a healthcare professional, fitness trainer, or celebrity. My credentials are simply that I'm an MMM: a middle-aged, menopausal mom.

I have more than 35 damn years of life experience, from the hormonal teenage years through pregnancy, motherhood, midlife crisis, and menopause. I have gained and lost weight throughout each stage and have received my share of painful battle scars along the way. I even gave up the endless, tortuous battle and cried.

This is my personal journey of weight loss, and after more than 50 years of living, gaining knowledge of what works and doesn't work, I am an expert regarding my personal health. I am also a little sassy. At this stage of life, I've earned the right to tell it like it is!

My Story

I began writing a personal journal to try to figure out why I was over 50 years old and was still obsessing, hyperventilating, and endlessly ranting and raving about my weight. I was a strong, hard-working, determined woman, yet I was failing miserably when it came to controlling my weight. Why?

I was also embarrassed and appalled that my whole world *still* revolved around food. Food became the devil and was always in control. I began to despise the words *diet* and *exercise*. I had become depressed, thinking it was all so hopeless, and I cried. I just cried.

After all those years searching for weight-loss answers from every possible source and trying most of the plans, I was still unsuccessful. I listened to all the experts and still found no plan that answered my specific needs. I looked around and realized that I was not alone. Hell, even some healthcare professionals are overweight.

I began my personal journal to theorize why I overate and then created a new game plan. I began by eliminating the negative words *diet* and *exercise* and replaced them with positive, fun phrases. I also found that through small changes I could gain more control, gain more calmness, and ultimately lose weight. I even had a little fun pretending the devil was responsible.

All I needed was laughter, common sense, and some easy, attainable personal goals. I became successful when I devised my own plan with simple strategies, including humor. I ultimately did it myself, without starvation diets or grueling, strenuous exercise. I learned that I didn't need to join a group or need someone to hold my hand.

My journey was about being kinder to myself. I've lived a half century and I've heard "no" too many times. I'm giving myself permission to add more yeses in my life.

I even discovered the most delicious chocolate cake recipe and found a way to include it into my life because I knew I couldn't possibly go through the rest of my life without the pleasure of the ultimate chocolate cake!

My personal weight-loss journey began by my believing I could be successful on my own. I started by telling all diet gurus, fitness experts, and skinny people to go to hell. Then I killed them, ate them, and still lost weight. You can, too.

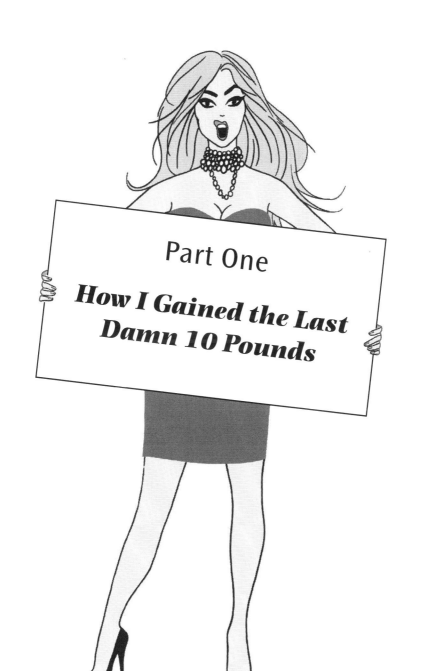

Part One

How I Gained the Last Damn 10 Pounds

Overview: Diet and Exercise Bullshit

Through my 50-plus years of living, I have listened to a lot of bullshit. I have witnessed people delivering it and people believing it. The weight-loss world is filled with it.

From the preachers with their miracle cures directly from God to the newest products and diet pills that will suppress hunger or even destroy those fat cells for us while we sleep, it's all bullshit. Bullshit, bullshit, and more bullshit. Every new discovery claims an even-more incredulous promise to get rid of fat.

Why do we keep buying into this BS? If there are so many diet programs, diet and exercise gurus, books, websites, diet-food packages, boot camps, weight-loss clinics, doctors, nutritionists, and dieticians, why are so many of us still overweight? Why do only a small percentage of us succeed, while some of us will succeed and then fail, and the rest of us will give up?

Because we don't want to accept our failures, we continue to believe in the diet and exercise BS. We look for newer and better products, hope for that scientific breakthrough, and pay big dollars for celebrity-endorsed products. The weight-loss industry knows this, and thus it continues the bullshit to make the diet world go round and round.

The weight-loss world is the perfect business. Since no program fits all and there is so much failure, there is a continual revolving client base, including new generations of overweight people willing to try something new. A never-ending client base means more profits, which leads to new products and gimmicks, which leads to more BS.

The saddest part of all of this is that most of us are so desperate to lose weight and get into better physical shape that we continue to try anything new, even if we know we are being set up to ultimately fail. Are we knowingly setting ourselves up to fail just to pretend we are in control and are not total losers? Do we knowingly accept the BS?

Maybe people aren't overweight because of fat; maybe we're just full of bullshit.

My personal journey through the maze of weight-loss endeavors is surely familiar to most of you. Please note that this is my journey: while the following are my failures, others have been successful with these endeavors.

- **Appetite suppressants.** In high school, I tried cheap appetite suppressants that actually tasted OK. I never found out if they were effective because I was a defiant teenager and eventually threw them out. No one was going to make me suppress my hunger and stop me from eating what I wanted and when. This same argument applies to me as an adult.
- **Aerobics classes.** These were fun at the beginning. The instructor was motivational, and the workouts weren't that strenuous. However, the logistics of going to the class several times a week became too much of a chore, and I resented the premise that I was paying to exercise. I soon ended the sessions.
- **Low-carb diet.** I wouldn't even consider this one. When given the choice between a piece of pizza or a steak, I'll go for the pizza. I'm definitely a carbs type of gal.

- **Weight-loss group.** Personal coaches sound wonderful. Having someone to encourage me and hold my hand while teaching me a healthier lifestyle was tempting, but also expensive. Plus, dietary restrictions left no room for the foods I really enjoy. Too many bland foods and portion sizes that were too small. Besides, I'm an adult. I know I have to eventually do this on my own.
- **Gym workouts.** I lack the passion to sustain a vigorous exercise regimen. I admit that I don't enjoy this type of workout.
- **Boot camps.** No way. If I don't have a passion for regular aerobic exercise, then I couldn't possibly endure this program.
- **Restrictive diets.** I tried these many times. Each time, I avoided favorite foods, such as pizza, potato chips, and chocolate, successfully for a few days, then, wham! I didn't just eat the forbidden foods, I gorged on them.
- **Diet pills.** I won't go there. I'm afraid of unknown side effects, and I don't trust drug companies' research.

My personal journey helped me wade through the weight-loss BS. I know that I will fail on most weight-loss plans because I'm not passionate about strenuous exercise, I don't enjoy most low-calorie meals, I won't use diet pills, and I won't totally restrict my diet. I also know that at this stage of my life someone holding my hand or guiding me is ridiculous. I know the real work begins when the group ends, the coaches go away, and you have to count calories and cook for yourself. The real battle begins after, without the "willpower in a box" to take home. The short-term fixes are over.

After all those years of attempts and failures, I know what doesn't work for me. I had to separate out all the diet and exercise bullshit and reexamine what is truthful, attainable, and, most important, sustainable concerning my personal wellbeing. I would no longer participate in the herd mentality. I would not sign up for a January 1st weight-loss and exercise program with the millions of others making New Year's resolutions that would be broken within months. I would no longer pretend to join a health club or gym. Gee, by ridding my life of this BS, I felt thinner already.

I began a new personal journey and tailor-made my plan. I rethought my perceptions of what diet and exercise really mean to me and I became successful. I did lose those last damn 10 pounds. You can, too.

1

Food Is the Devil

I read a book claiming that sugar is the devil, and I disagree. *All* food is the devil, every single morsel.

How can food be the devil? Fifty-plus years have shown me that as a mortal, I am not strong enough to stand up to my never-ending cravings and wishes, which, of course, are masterminded by the devil. We are enticed by food's appearance, lured by its aromas, and intoxicated by its flavors. What seduction and pleasure! The devil is the ultimate marketer.

In the end, we are betrayed by the devil, and then we must face the consequence of our overindulgences: weight gain. It's a painful consequence because the weight gain consists of fat bulges, ridges, cellulose, and extra weight to carry around. It's painful because these fat cells are not evenly distributed. Some of us get fat thighs, pudgy faces, fat stomachs, or fat butts. We turn into caricatures of ourselves. Painful, because our enlarged body parts are on public display. Painful because we know our emotional wellbeing has been messed with.

Painful because the devil is around every corner, trying to sabotage our fight against this fat buildup.

The moment that I knew food was the devil occurred when I was on my last and final diet. My family was eating my favorite comfort food for dinner: pizza. I stoically declined a slice, not because of the calories but because one slice would never satisfy me. You see, I might as well call pizza *pig-za*, because I can't control myself. That night while my family was asleep and I was watching TV, I noticed myself staying up later and later. At about 1 A.M., I somehow lost all of my senses and convinced myself that I was now entitled to a slice of pizza because it was, after all, a new day. No longer in control of my mental faculties, I marched straight to the refrigerator. Did I have a lapse in judgment? A psychotic episode? Or was I possessed by the devil, who finally got his way?

The devil is tricky and persistent. We can't go anywhere without having food in one hand and a drink in the other, just as the devil planned. Think about it: everywhere you go, no matter what time of day you'll see someone munching or slurping. Drivers, walkers, students, workers, young kids, even churchgoers are partaking in non-stop eating and drinking. Yes, the devil even follows us into church during those divine services.

In fact, the devil has you convinced that it's God's will to celebrate every momentous occasion of your life, even your death, with food. Every blessed event of your life from the day you are born until the day you die will center on food.

Before you are born everyone is already celebrating your anticipated arrival with that adorable baby-themed cake created for your baby shower. Imagine that, people are celebrating you but are starting without you. They couldn't even wait until you arrived. It was all about the cake. After you arrive, they'll again enjoy eating cake while they laugh (at your expense) as you create cake art all over your face. The devil doesn't make kids an exception.

At your funeral, you'll have to worry about someone spilling crumbs on you in your casket. People are once again thinking about you as they eat food without you. We can't even say goodbye to our loved ones without food playing a major role. Mourners will cry, cry, cry . . . and off they go to the after-funeral buffet.

The devil is always prompting us. One of his biggest weapons is desserts. The dessert promises a return to our youth; at least according to you know who, we're magically transformed into kids again. Desserts are fun, yummy, and decadent. Just look at how big your eyes get when you first see the dessert presentation—wide open and blazing, just like the devil's.

What about that devil's sense of humor? Picture all those brides and grooms on their wedding day, smashing their wedding cake into each other's faces. Wedding couples surrounded by friends and family suddenly losing control and lunging at each other with pieces of their special cake. And the messier the cake fight, the better! At first we're horrified. Then everyone laughs and encourages the newlyweds. Hmmm. . . . What really happened? Was this wedding tradition created by humans, or is the devil having fun at our expense?

Some people blame marketing. After all, we have all had incredible food dreams due to late-night commercials, leading us to make unwise food decisions the next day. But, no, I blame it on the devil. Marketers couldn't possibly hold that much power over us. Definitely the workings of the devil, and he is frighteningly everywhere.

If every morsel of food is the devil, and the devil is so determined to make us fat and keep us fat, what is a poor mortal to do? Through our own personal journeys, we can explore our weaknesses regarding food and exercise, knowing that there will be days when we will say, "Who gives a damn? I am going to eat that whole chocolate cake!" What you can do is create your own journey, as I have, to focus your strengths and minimize your weaknesses. We may not beat the devil, but we can certainly outmaneuver him more often than not.

2

The Aha! Moment:
Why I Overeat

I can't control myself, I can't control myself, I just can't control myself when it comes to food. Help!

Actually, food is the one thing that I can control in my life, and that's why I was overweight. It took me many years to realize how profound this statement is:

I overeat because it is the only thing I can control in my life.

It is as simple as that. This was the "Aha!" moment I had been searching for. I would eat when I wanted, what I wanted, and how much I wanted *because I could.*

When I was feeling frustrated about something, I would have pizza *because I could.*

If I was feeling lonely, I would have an ice cream sundae to comfort me *because I could.*

I would skip exercise for no good reason and eat whatever I wanted *because I could.*

When my dog George died, I cried for three days straight and still chose to overeat *because I could.*

After a great day, I would have two pieces of cake to celebrate *because I could.*

In other words, I was blaming overeating on disappointment, loneliness, laziness, heartbreak, even joy. I am an adult. I know when I'm feeling each one of these emotions. I know the correct behavioral response to each. I know eating couldn't possibly be the right response to any of these emotions. Yet I still chose food instead of dealing with the underlying emotion. Eating was the only part of my life where someone else dared not interfere.

For goodness' sake, even a child knows you're offering him a cookie to try to make him feel better because his friend won't play with him.

I overeat because I can.

We are all searching for that one underlying problem that we harbor and that makes us overeat. As if one childhood problem or one adult problem or one traumatic experience makes us resort to excessive eating over and over. One problem? With all the uncertainties in life, with all the things we can't control, it seems to me that we have many excuses we can use to overeat, not just one. And, unfortunately, the uncertainties continue throughout our lives.

Please note
I am not a psychologist or a physician. I have also never endured a truly traumatic event. Yes, the loss of my dog was terribly sad for me; yet I know that there are worse tragedies that I will face in my lifetime and that others have already faced. For those who have and who are

truly self-medicating with food, I hope you get the professional help that you need.

The rest of us need to learn how to get a better grip on our behavioral responses. Just because we can't indulge our fantasies when dealing with injustices (such as punching a horrible boss, slapping a belligerent relative, or running over the neighbor's barking dog) doesn't mean we should use food as our salvation. We may not be able to control the injustice, but we can certainly control our responses.

The phrase *emotional eater* is overused. I hear it so often that it feels like an excuse. "I overeat because I am always so emotional about everything." "If I wasn't so emotional, I wouldn't eat so much." I've heard lots of these statements. Studies show that the reason many people gain weight and keep it on is due to this emotional eating. Maybe we can't control our every emotion, but we can control every piece of food that enters our mouths. We overeat because we feel powerless and we can control eating.

Immediately after you've overindulged in food, do you feel guilty? You should. You have just engaged in an inappropriate behavior, a behavior that you chose, a behavior that you can control.

The next time you're feeling an emotion that leads you to pick up something to eat, ask yourself whether the food item will really make you feel better about the situation or whether it will just make you feel as if you have temporarily gained power over the situation. If you find yourself grabbing any food item in sight just to eat something, you are definitely using food to control your situation. This is what I was doing. I seldom found pleasure in the foods I chose at those moments because I was either fuming over the situation or zoning out, trying to forget the ordeal. It was a temporary fix, with my control over the food giving me my power back. (That devil with his mind games is incorrigible!)

My personal "Aha!" moment has been life changing for me. I recognized that I wasn't trying to make myself feel better through food gratification; I was overeating to control the outcome. I never enjoyed the food, I enjoyed the power it gave me. I overate because I could.

3

Who the Hell Wants to Be Skinny?

orget the "skinny girl" goal here. *Skinny* means thin or emaciated, which translates to not normal. Skinny belongs to the foolish young girls who are trying to maintain today's youthful celebrity looks. It's unrealistic. Remind yourself of the few actresses who have been known to be slightly anorexic. Icky! Rib bones and hip bones are not attractive.

Even the current celebrity weight-loss endorsers are not aiming for a skinny body. They are after a "healthy weight." They are cautious not to promise impossible weight-loss goals because chances are they aren't reachable and, more important, even if they are, they can't be maintained.

Another current trend in diet books is skinny this and thin that. Have you actually read those books and tried their eating plans? One book wants you to become a complete vegan. No meat, chicken, fish, or dairy products. Fasting regularly is also recommended.

To me, this is such an extreme lifestyle change that I can't even contemplate it. This plan totally removes all food pleasures for me. I have yet to find a true dietetic replacement for my delicious chocolate cake recipe.

Another book wants you to graze instead of eating your complete meal, ordering appetizers and side dishes and taking nibbles only. Imagine your entire life eating this way—tasting food sparingly, searching for non-calorie foods to fill up on. Those aren't meals; they're not even hors d'oeuvres. It seems like extreme torture to me. And I'm mortified to think that I could only have a few bites of my scrumptious chocolate cake.

In all fairness, these books are filled with lots of research, information, and personal experience. One book claims that sugar is the devil. I partially agree, because all food is the devil. Both types of books want you to eat real foods (foods that are not processed), and maybe eating less meat is a good idea since meat is harder for our digestive systems to process. I learned from these books, but I also found that they call for extreme measures. Their way of eating reminds me of survival-mode living, in which you eat only enough to sustain your life. Read these books and judge for yourself if these plans are for you. Personally, if you take away so many of my food pleasures, I will become one homicidal woman. Maybe that is why some of these book authors use so much profanity.

Take note, too, who writes these books. Some are former models. Their point of view is from living in a skinny world. This may be hard for most of us to relate to. Some are under the age of 40 and have not experienced hormonal and metabolism changes. Others have not even experienced pregnancy and motherhood and the effects of those significant changes on your body. What could you possibly know about dieting if you haven't experienced the three biggest factors that attribute to weight gain in women: being pregnant, being a mother, and experiencing metabolism changes after 40?

The physical process of being pregnant brings hormonal changes to your body. You may experience cravings that lead to extra pounds, or you may gain extra weight because you feel the need to eat for two.

Becoming a mother presents other challenges that may result in weight gain. You are now responsible for another human being, who at the moment is extremely helpless and fragile. Your emotions will run the gamut, from euphoria to panic, with everything in between. All this emotional stuff is pretty stressful and may lead you to the refrigerator for comfort, because, for most of us, there is little or no outside help.

As we age, several factors influence our metabolism that may make it harder to lose weight after the age of 40. One of these factors is muscle mass. If we slow down or reduce our physical activities as we age, we will burn fewer calories because of reduced muscle mass. It is important to maintain physical activity as we age and not buy into society's portrayal of retirement as an easy lifestyle and a time to slow down.

If you haven't experienced all of these factors, don't even pretend to know a damn thing about weight gain and weight loss. Please, just go away and eat your half of a celery stick.

The last damn 10 pounds don't mean those pounds that will make your butt so tiny that you will have to buy padded underwear to give you curves. They don't mean being skinny. The last damn 10 pounds mean getting to whatever your individual acceptable weight should be and whatever you can maintain.

4

Shut Up, Celebrity Weight-Loss Endorsers!

Unless you are such a fan of a celebrity that you would follow his or her advice no matter what, stop paying attention to celebrity weight-loss endorsers.

This was one of the biggest reasons that I knew I was on my own to lose weight. I, too, watched celebrities lose weight as spokespersons for weight-loss programs. I cheered them on and congratulated them as they succeeded with everyone else who was watching. Wow. They had lost weight and now it was my turn.

I bought into it and prayed that I'd be able to follow the celebrities' plans. But then reality smacked me in my commoner face, and I had to admit that celebrities don't represent me and never will. How could they? While the rest of us are juggling full-time schedules that include working, taking care of kids, running our households, and, the hardest job of all, being emotional cheerleaders for our families and ourselves, celebrities have the opportunity to hire people to do these things for them. Some are even part-time parents and spouses at best. Being a rich celebrity gives one access to help that the rest of us can only dream about, and I'm not talking about the diet counselors on these programs, either. Big deal! These celebrity weight-loss endorsers have access to an entire staff to help them lose weight: personal trainer, nutritionist, nanny, personal assistant, personal secretary, maid, chef, driver, dog walker, school tutor, fans to boost the ego, and a spouse who comes with his own entourage of help so he isn't infringing on the celebrity's time with his problems. And of course, there's a manager to direct them all and find the celebrity new and interesting projects on top of all this.

Celebrities also have the emotional support that is so important to losing weight. The rest of us have to fight this battle of self-encouragement by ourselves, every single moment. It takes an army of strength to stop that devil, who is always discouraging us and tempting us. And let's not forget that fat endorsement check. (Attention national weight-loss centers: throw money at me and I will show you real bones, real fast!)

The real kick is that some of these celebrity endorsers don't get close to losing the last 10 pounds, and they don't even claim to have this as their goal. They all want to be healthier or whatever their personal tagline is. Plus, they get national TV exposure. Public encouragement and ridicule are strong enticements for celebrities. It is almost a last-ditch approach to weight loss for them.

Remember that this is a job for the celebrities. They are paid to be spokespeople so it is in their best interest to lose weight. The rest of us have to work this into our busy lives without the monetary incentive. In fact, we have to pay if we want to be part of these weight-loss programs.

The ultimate tragedy is that some of the celebrities got fat again.

I'm officially signing off from paying attention to celebrities on this issue. Maybe you should, too.

5

Are Medical Professionals Ignoring Their Own Advice?

I don't mean to be a bitch; I'm just frustrated beyond belief. Enough is enough. After a half century of life experience, I feel I'm entitled to say it like it is.

Have you been to a medical center lately? If you haven't, take a field trip to see all the plump doctors, nurses, and even nutritionists, because I must be missing something. Is it suddenly acceptable to be 20, 30, or more pounds overweight? These overweight professionals are counseling us?

Let me clarify something: I respect doctors and nurses. They give a damn about other human beings, and they know exactly what life they have chosen. Every day they see, hear, touch, and smell things that I don't even want to know about. They see frightened human beings. They see lots of suffering and desperation. They see terror on parents' faces. They even see humans begging to die. Let me repeat: doctors and nurses give a damn about other human beings. Maybe it's OK for them to eat a few more sweets to compensate for the life they have chosen.

Maybe it's OK if we all self-medicate with food. Because, after all, life is fragile. But wait, these are the medical superheroes. If they can't help themselves, we're all doomed.

This chapter is a reality check to you and me to once again show that we are really alone in this journey. Everywhere you look, no matter what profession one has chosen, we all face this fat issue, and there is no definitive answer. We have to find this one out for ourselves.

Self-Love Fest

I love myself, I love myself, I really do love myself. So why the hell do I still overeat?

The latest diet fad is all about self-love and food. Really, this is just another series of long, boring diet books. If you love yourself, then you will stop overeating. You're kidding, right? I don't buy into the theory that if you love yourself, all will be well.

Remember in an earlier chapter when I realized that I overeat because I can? This applies whether I'm happy with my life or I think life sucks. Some days I love myself, other days I'm not so sure about this self-love deal. I am an emotional being with ups and downs. It doesn't matter if I am giving myself a high five or chastising myself. I overeat because I can. It is one of the few things I can control in my life.

Why are we making this so hard?

Along with books that teach self-love as a method to help you from overeating, there are retreats that focus on this subject, held in beautiful, peaceful settings, far from your everyday, stress-filled life.

Everyone holds hands and sings "Kumbaya." After a few days of listening to spiritual gurus talking gently to you about self-love in a calm, natural setting, you'll swear that you have found inner peace. That is what retreats are for: rejuvenating your soul. And with your spirit full, you say goodbye as the gurus symbolically release you, proclaiming that since your spirit is full, your stomach doesn't have to be. You are certain that your new-found self-love is permanent, as you were given self-help books and materials to bring home with you to keep the spiritual journey on track.

This touchy-feely spiritual crap lasts as long as you can keep yourself in a retreat-type trance, most likely until something or someone irritates you. It's no different than returning from vacation: all is well until you enter your real life again. As you return to your old routines, the foggy trance starts to dissipate and unpleasantness begins to surround you. You keep the self-love thing going until . . . the moment when the unpleasant hits you in your face. Your dog barks at you to take him outside—pronto—and it's raining. Not now, Fido. Can't you wait until it stops raining? The dog barks louder and starts pacing frantically. You scramble to reread your retreat information, chanting over and over in your head how much you love yourself. The dog looks at you for the fool you are and barks even louder. You throw the book at the dog.

Gone is the peace, gone is the self-love. The trance is over. You must take the dog outside now and face the reality that you will have one soggy dog to take care of later. After you reenter the house and dry off the dog, you run to your secret chocolate stash and chow down every last piece to get back to your "happy" place.

Your gurus forgot to tell you that self-love is an everyday process and that you are not on this journey alone. More important, they forgot to mention that everyone around you (including your dog) needs to love themselves and you too, or the whole Kumbaya thing fails.

Why do we make life so difficult? When did we lose our common sense? Of course we should love ourselves. Of course we should be kind to ourselves. Of course we should forgive ourselves. Of course we shouldn't self-medicate ourselves with food.

Of course we shouldn't overeat because we can.

7

God, Please Help Us . . .

If the devil is responsible for our bad food behavior, where is God? Why isn't he helping us? Surely millions of us pray every day, yet we keep getting fatter. Why aren't our prayers getting answered? Why can't we pray ourselves thin?

God gave humans the intelligence to know what to do and what not to do concerning our general health. We unequivocally know how we gain weight: we eat more calories than we burn off. He also gave us the willpower needed to keep us from eating out of control. Some of us just can't do it. Again, does the devil always win?

- Child: learns the difference between good behavior and bad behavior
- Adult: experiments with good and bad behaviors
- Mature adult: chooses behaviors

How does this relate to our food choices?

As children we learn which behaviors will earn us rewards and which will earn us punishments, and we act accordingly. Our food decisions may not be our own, but we learn quickly that good behavior will result in cookies or ice cream and bad behavior may result in no dessert after dinner.

As adults, we may exhibit both behaviors. We may eat sparingly at an event, or we may gorge ourselves at the buffet. We may eat modestly while on a date, and then eat ravenously when we arrive home. We experiment with foods and exercise to see what works, either incorporating them into our lifestyle or skipping them. We will lie to everyone, including our doctors, about how much we exercise. We will lie about what types of foods we eat and how much we drink. We will lie about it all. At this stage we still believe we can get away with our tiny lies. We even pray to God to at least make our friends fat, too, if he isn't going to make us thin.

As mature adults, we choose our behaviors based on life experiences. We make conscious decisions based on truths. We know that overeating is bad food behavior, but we choose it anyhow. Afterwards, we know what we've done, but some of us may still pray to God for some type of miracle to reverse our poor behavior.

We know it is our choice to overeat. God gave us this knowledge and he gave us the willpower to stop overeating. We just choose not to. We make excuses, we lie to ourselves, and we look for manmade miracles in every new diet book or fad diet. God has always been with us; we choose to ignore him because his path for us does not end with a chocolate chip cookie. We choose to believe the promise of foolish men and women instead of God.

God will not silence the devil among us foolish humans. It is our choice alone to act foolishly or not. God will not do the work for us, no matter how hard we pray. He will let the devil win.

8

Shut Up, or I Will Kill You and Then Eat You!

ecall all the diet and exercise start-ups and subsequent failures you've had. How many were based on the newest diet book or fad? How many friends joined you? Which fitness clubs did you join? Which diet organizations did you join?

Sorry, but you will be in this endeavor alone. No matter how many friends or groups you join, you will ultimately be responsible for yourself. Everyone cheats. Belonging to a group will not stop you from scheming and strategizing when you want to sneak that forbidden candy bar.

I remember working at a company where the receptionist, whose desk was situated for all to see, was successfully losing weight. Her goal was to be a healthier weight before becoming pregnant. As this overweight gal began to noticeably slim down, she had the entire company rooting for her. How great was that? Maybe too great, because as I was walking down the street to our second office building one day, I saw her eating an ice cream cone. When she saw me, her red face said it all—she was busted. Family, friends, and coworkers weren't enough to keep her from even a temporary loss of willpower. She alone had to do all the work.

I tried getting my family involved in helping me. I made paper caricatures of big butts and put them all over the kitchen walls and cupboards. For each pound lost, I would take down one butt. My kids and husband thought this was hilarious at first, but they soon challenged my mental state to have to resort to such a tactic. Alas, this desperate endeavor failed.

And gals, forget about dieting with your husband or boyfriend. Somehow all of my friends' guys could easily lose those few extra pounds. It's as if it were just a simple chore for them to do. My husband is the same, only supercharged. When he exercises, he goes full out, and he applies the same determination to dieting. He does all the right stuff. Sure, I'm proud of him, but when we attempted to lose weight together, it became obvious that he was more committed and was kicking my butt. Seeing my failure, he proceeded to tell me his philosophies and to lecture me on strategies, blah, blah, blah. I told him, "Good for you! Now SHUT UP, OR I WILL KILL YOU AND THEN EAT YOU!"

Beware of She-Devils

 $\mathcal{S}$ tay away from she-devils. You know, bitchy women who don't want you as a friend because they think you are the competition. They converse with you while staring up and down at your body. They don't care about the conversation, they are only checking you out and comparing themselves to you.

You can identify these women immediately through their facial expressions. Instead of smiling at you, they squint at you, looking for your every flaw. These women don't even realize how obvious they are. They will never be friends with you or give you needed advice. But they will be all too eager to give you hurtful advice that you don't want or need.

Most women are so trusting that we don't want to believe that a sister would deliberately betray us. But she-devils will.

Remember your group of girlfriends in high school? How many times do you think they gave you compliments to your face when they were secretly laughing at you? Chances are, more than you think, and you were probably doing the same to them. Jealousy and meanness are a big part of our society.

People are also very uncomfortable with telling the truth. I can recall only one friend who confided to me that she was worried that I was gaining weight. It was during my senior year of high school and I had gained several pounds. My girlfriend told me point-blank that I had gained the notorious senior spread of 10 to 15 pounds. At first I was shocked because this girlfriend bordered on being a mean girl. You were careful around her because she was one of the queen bees. Her social status could influence whether you would be invited to the next great party or not. Her sharp tongue made many girls cry. So was she being kind because she cared or mean because that was her personality? Surely, my other, kinder friends would tell me the truth.

They did not. Lie after lie came from them. No one backed her up. My other friends couldn't or wouldn't tell me the truth. Even though they were kind, gentle girls who would not purposely hurt my feelings, they hurt me by telling those little white lies. They let me believe I was fine when I had a problem. Girlfriend after girlfriend told me how great I looked and that, in fact, they were the ones who need to lose a few pounds. It turns out that this queen bee was actually doing me a favor. She told me like it was: I was overweight. I took notice and I owned up to it.

Adult friends are no different. Rarely do you make a connection with someone whom you can comfortably be honest with. People are notorious for changing the subject when it comes to giving an honest opinion on a personal subject. If they do, it could turn confrontational. It is better to sugarcoat things than to start a heated conversation. Just watch one of the current reality shows featuring housewives.

What a perfect example of a woman's ability to look someone straight in the face and lie. Watch how they greet each other. The first words out of their mouths are how nice each other looks while they are giving each other a big hug and kiss. Later in the show, their claws and sharp tongues come out and no one looks pretty anymore. It seems everyone lies, mostly about weight. Look in the mirror and hop on that scale. See the truth for yourself.

Family can be toxic, too. While visiting a relative, I mentioned how we had each gained a few pounds (my relative had actually gained a lot) and how we should work on losing them. My relative angrily yelled at me to accept my body as it was because her doctor told her that her weight was fine. What? I was confiding in her about both of our weight gains, hoping that she would commiserate with me, but she chose to be high and mighty and blame me for thinking it was a problem. She was lecturing me on body image when in fact she had just fabricated an outrageous excuse, pretending it had come from her doctor. How is that for a toxic response from the ultimate she-devil?

Surround yourself with caring, nurturing female friends. You know, the gals who will laugh and joke with you about anything. The gals who will gently tell you the truth. The gals who will help you with your personal weight-loss journey while keeping all the details private. Banish all those she-devils from your life. Give them a 20-pound box of stale chocolates as a parting gift.

10

Gals: Stop Being Diet Fools

Gals, be careful when evaluating diet plans. We buy the majority of diet books and products, so marketers are targeting us. Beware of marketers trying to sell you rapid–weight-loss products and plans due to research finding that men may have the ability to lose weight faster than women. There are numerous plans that claim miraculous results.

Men and women burn calories differently, and a major reason for this is hormones. Research has shown that the male hormone testosterone enables men to have more muscle and less fat. Having a higher percentage of muscle works to men's advantage: it allows them to eat more because muscle burns more calories than fat. A man who engages in moderate activity can eat between 2,200 and 2,800 calories a day, depending on his age. Women, on the other hand, produce estrogen for childbearing, which causes them to store more fat, needed to nourish the fetus and to later breastfeed the baby. A moderately active woman needs between 1,800 and 2,200 calories per day, depending on her age.

As women approach menopause, they encounter new challenges. Fat once stored in their hips, thighs, and butts redistributes to their middles. Estrogen levels diminish, causing the body to search for other sources of estrogen. Unfortunately, another source of estrogen is fat cells, so the body learns to convert more calories to fat to increase estrogen production. This means weight gain and that dreaded "middle-age spread." About 90 percent of women between the ages of 35 and 50 gain an average of 10 to 15 pounds, and it mostly appears around the middle area.

Other research shows that men are able to lose weight through increased exercise alone. For women, the extra fat produced by estrogen may not go away with exercise alone. Dietary changes—specifically, eating less fat—produces more weight loss than changes in exercise. Thus, women have to work harder to lose weight through both diet and exercise due to hormones. Remember that plans for rapid weight loss may give immediate results, but you are not resolving your long-term health needs. These plans do not address the hormone issue.

Sure, men have great ideas on weight loss, but until they experience female hormones and changes due to childbirth and menopause, I don't want to listen to them. As much I respect medically trained males giving diet advice, they are still men. It is their wives and girlfriends I want to talk to. They are the ones to help me with those chocolate cravings. Men can tell me all the medical explanations frontwards and backwards, but they can't stop that she-devil in me screaming, "Kill all men trying to stop you from eating that chocolate! And for a bonus, eat them, too!"

11

Gluttony Breaks One of the Ten Commandments

*L*ife is not one giant smorgasbord. There is a reason that "Thou shalt not be a glutton" is one of God's Ten Commandments. OK, it's not, but it should be.

Everyone loves chubby-faced babies sent from heaven above. But for crying out loud, those babies had better start their crawling marathons and lose that baby fat ASAP. Chubby babies are cute, overweight children are not.

I am currently raising two girls who are now in their teens. As a parent, I was responsible for monitoring their eating habits and exercise when they were young, and I took this responsibility seriously. If my kids ate too much junk food, it was my fault. If my kids did not try new foods, it was my fault. If my kids did not learn how to ride a bike, swim, hike, or play outside, again it was my fault. If my kids did not hear the word *no* or ever use it themselves, it was certainly my fault. Sure, I made mistakes. Of course I overindulged them. The point is that I am proud that my teenagers are thriving and have good body images, and it would have been completely my fault if I had let my kids overeat and not exercise.

When we see an overweight child, we think lazy and uninformed parents, and in most cases we're right. Do not sugarcoat this. Parents are lazy when they choose food gratification over their kids' wellbeing. Not being able to say no means you are failing as a parent. Do you think your children are happy that their own parents keep making them heavier? Sadly, no one looks at an overweight child and believes it is just a phase that they will grow out of. No one! All we see is an overweight kid who will be an overweight teen, who will ultimately become an overweight adult. Parents, please try harder.

This applies to pets also. Don't show your dogs or cats how much you love them through food. I think we've all seen a dog that was so obese that it actually waddled. Everyone, from strangers to veterinarians, tried to persuade the owners to stop loving their dog so much, but they ignored the advice. They didn't care about their dog's health but about how good they felt by spoiling their pet. Too bad their dog couldn't bark back, "Bad owners! Bad owners!"

There are difficult obstacles we all have to face:

- **Life is not a giant smorgasbord.** We can't eat second helpings just for the sake of eating.
- **Fast-food cravings will get you.** Know what your cravings are and control them by incorporating them into your plan.
- **Food portions are huge.** When it comes to food and human behavior, humans are undeniably simpletons. We see big portions, and we show smiles; we see skimpy portions, and we show teeth. Restaurants know this. They also know that you will

supersize anything for a few pennies or a dollar more. Face it, the food industry is encouraging you to overeat for just a few pennies more. Especially help your kids here. What would you do if your kids offered you 50 cents from their allowance to supersize their dinner?

- **The devil plays the guilt card on us.** The devil will pressure us to eat everything on our plates because of the poor, starving children in the world. This one always works.
- **People who lived through the Great Depression won't waste food.** You are expected to eat every last bite. Right now. Even if you are full.

Life is not one giant smorgasbord. Let's make this the Eleventh Commandment.

12

A Skinny World

*M*odels do not represent 99 percent of women. Most of us are average looking, with meat on our bones, and we accept it. An average woman in America weighs almost 165 pounds. Models with real-world bodies are gaining more advertising space, but not fast enough. In fact, skinny models under the age of 16 are actually gaining popularity on the runway. Should this be happening?

Models play an important role in fashion merchandising. We love the glamour and fantasy they invoke. But models achieve superstar status and earn big bucks for being young, attractive, and thin. Is bestowing celebrity status on thin models creating good role models for women? Should we worry that our daughters might idolize them and have poor body images if they can't achieve this status? Should we worry that our daughters might try drastic dieting measures to try to be size zero?

Let's help our teens see skinny models for who they are. Most have ectomorph body types; they're tall and thin. Most women are endomorphs, people with pear shapes or round bodies. No amount of dieting or exercise will make endomorphs into ectomorphs. The modeling world is also filled with deceptive airbrushing, plastic surgery, and computer imaging. In the real world, we can't airbrush away our imperfections.

Our hopes and goals for teenage girls should include personal empowerment. One way girls can obtain this is by participating in sports. Look at middle schools and high schools: not only do girls enjoy sports but they also want in on the college sports scholarships. Where cheerleading and dance squads once ruled because of their glamorous aspect, they now get greater respect as a result of their competitiveness. They are no longer classified as pretty-face competitions. Talent and athleticism are now required, which require strong, healthy bodies and minds.

Girls haven't given up their interest in fashion and glamour; in fact, I'm sure they want it all. Just not at a skinny size, we hope.

13

To Hell with Dieting, Just Throw Money at the Problem!

No kidding, dieting is hard. When you reach the "what should I try now?" plateau and don't want to diet and exercise the old-fashioned way, what are your options?

- Join that weight-loss group with the celebrity spokesperson.
- Enroll in an exercise program.
- Take diet pills.
- Hire a professional trainer.
- Hire a professional nutritionist.
- Buy the latest best-selling diet book and follow it.
- Buy several diet books and follow them all.
- Get liposuction.
- Purchase store-bought packaged diet foods.
- Go on a crash diet.
- Take appetite suppressants.

- Get breast implants; even women will ignore your fat body and stare only at your gigantic breasts.
- Try hypnosis.

Try one, try them all. See if throwing money at the problem will make the fat go away. Pay someone to lead you, guide you, torture you, even trick you—whatever you think you need to accomplish your goal. In other words, do your own research and then follow the advice that seems compatible with your strengths and personality. Do this once and for all to see if one of these methods will actually work. Remember, though, you must think long-term here. Most of these are temporary plans for jump-starting your weight loss.

If you're one of the lucky few who succeeds with one of these methods, great! If not, you know for yourself what works for you and what doesn't.

For the approximately 95 percent of you who will not succeed long term with any of the above, join me in telling all diet gurus, fitness experts, and skinny people to go to hell. Now let's kill them, eat them, and still lose weight.

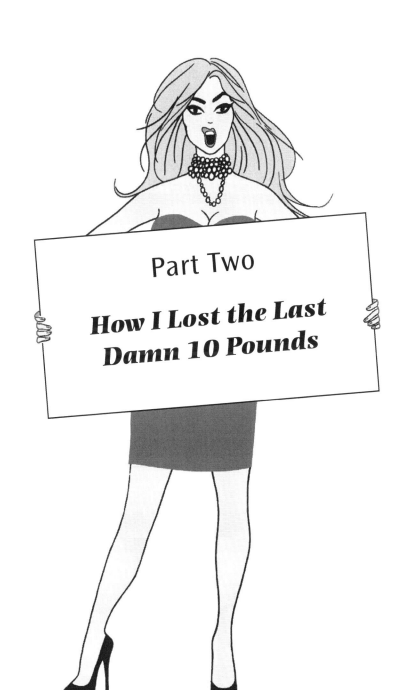

Part Two

How I Lost the Last
Damn 10 Pounds

Overview: Create Your Own Personal Journal

Let's help ourselves. Let's change our lifestyles gradually so that we can regain control of our lives, be healthier, and ultimately be happier. Let's create our own personalized journals incorporating a simple five-step plan that will help us lose those last damn 10, 15, 20 . . . pounds.

The five steps that we will discuss in detail in Part Two are:

1. **Laugh:** Let's add laughter and humor to our lives where diet and exercise are concerned. Our goal is to replace negative, self-defeating attitudes with positive, encouraging ones. We don't want diet gurus humiliating us into following impossible restrictive and survival-type food plans. We also don't want to be bullied or tortured during exercise to achieve results. Most important, we don't need skinny people yelling obscenities at us. We can change our lifestyles through positive, even funny tactics and strategies.

2. **Take baby steps:** Making small changes will give us control, help us destress our lives, and give us greater confidence. Each baby step we take and accomplish will lead us closer to our goals and success.

3. **Create strategies:** I'll outline specific strategies for lifestyle changes, including a new philosophy on eating patterns that is gaining national attention. I'll also discuss a new game plan for exercise.

4. **Learn the secrets:** I'll reveal secrets that will help us avoid the many pitfalls that dieters face.
5. **Follow the words of wisdom:** These words of wisdom will help us guide our kids, prepare us for restaurant excursions, and help us with everyday living.

This five-step plan was created from my 35-plus years of real-life experiences. As you create your own personal journal, incorporate the knowledge gained through your life experiences. Be honest, as I have been about my own, regarding what your strengths and weaknesses are. Then use your strengths and a positive attitude to work toward your goals.

This is not a one-size-fits-all plan. The purpose of this book is for you to discover what works for you, just as I did. Remember that permanent change takes time, and each of us will find our "Aha!" moments at different stages. For example, choosing a new word for *diet* may be easy for some, but others may take longer to erase the word from their vocabulary.

So, begin with **laughter**, **take baby steps** to build confidence, follow some **strategies** using **secrets** and **words of wisdom**, and begin your personal journey.

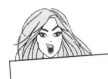

14

Laugh

*A*re you choosing to go through life as a crabby old person or a loveable old soul? Be the loveable old soul and laugh.

Let's stare at our bodies, analyze our features, and have a really good laugh, because bodies are strange and often funny looking.

All bodies—whether young or old, good-looking or not—have body parts that look peculiar. Our ears protrude out of the sides of our heads, our noses protrude from the front of our faces, our heads swivel in most directions and even bob up and down. Our eyes can look angelic or devilish; they can even look at each other! Our arms swing while we walk. We also have odd-looking joints and protruding bones from our wrists, ankles, and collarbones.

As we age, our ears, nose, and feet continue to grow. How hilarious! Our skin wrinkles and sags, our joints make cracking sounds, and our minds lose focus, causing us to repeat our stories. We even have a harder time controlling our flatulence. And we're worried about our weight?

Let's bring laughter into our lives to help us deal with the aging process and how it may cause fluctuations in our weight. Let's laugh at all the ridiculous goals we've envisioned for ourselves, including unrealistic weight loss to get to that perfect weight.

Let's laugh about how absurd the diet industry has become. The nation has become so obsessed with weight loss that grueling boot-camp workouts in which participants are bullied to hyper-exercise and eat starvation-type rations has become our primetime TV. Fat celebrities are going on national TV to endorse weight-loss plans. There are TV shows about obese people getting gastric bypass surgery for weight loss. The nation views these types of shows as entertainment!

For those of us who are not primetime TV material, laughter will help us on our weight-loss journey. Laughter will help us by giving us the positive energy needed to begin our journey, to overcome the setbacks and disappointments that may occur, to become successful, and to help us maintain our success.

15

Choose a Secret Reason to Lose Weight

*E*mpower yourself. *Select a reason to lose weight:*

- My sex life will be better.
- I will be happy.
- I won't have to bleach the crap out of my hair to distract the attention away from my flab.
- I will be free to overindulge again.
- I will attract a new sugar daddy or sugar momma.
- I will be discovered.
- I will be able to keep up the pace walking my dog without my hips knocking him over.
- I will make my ex jealous because once I am thin, I will obviously be a wild thing in bed.
- I will shut up that nagging relative/friend.
- I will fit into my skinny jeans and steal my teenager's boyfriend/girlfriend.

- I will look like a Barbie or Ken doll, and the whole world will adore me.
- I will look my wedding-day best; I just have to look better than that one female guest who shows up at every wedding, trying to steal the spotlight by being inappropriately dressed and acting like a sex goddess.
- I will fit on the back of that Harley motorcycle.
- I will be able to start living my life.
- I will become rich and famous.
- I will be youthful again.
- I will write the next bestseller diet book.
- I will write the next coffee table sex book and my picture will be on the cover.

Wasn't that fun! Now forget about them. The real reason you are trying to lose weight is to:

- a. Silence the devil.
- b. Make your body and mind function better.
- c. Laugh more.
- d. All of the above.

The correct answer is d. All of the above.

16.

Die, Diet, Die!

I am going to create a new national holiday. Every January 1 will now be:

FFD Day, or Freedom From Dieting Day

No more New Year's Day diet resolutions. No more proclaiming that on this day I am going to begin my diet. No more impossible goals. No more empty promises. No more justifying eating like a pig throughout the holiday season because you will start that infamous New Year's diet. No more joining a fitness program or gym in January, only to stop going after two or three months. Stop. Just stop. Die, diet, die. This New Year's resolution has to end.

I would like to be in Times Square on New Year's Eve. After the moment everyone shouts, "Happy New Year!" I want to scream, "NO MORE DIET RESOLUTIONS!"

Let's face reality. Diets don't work. They suck. We even despise the word *diet*. Most important, each of us is in diet hell because of it, feeling like we will never get out. This repetition of dieting as a New Year's resolution year after year must end.

Let's replace it with kinder, more manageable resolutions that we will look forward to. Let's keep New Year's Day as the rejuvenation time that it should be: a happy, peaceful new beginning, not the same old drudgery of trying to redeem ourselves from our fat sins year after year.

We need to ultimately change the way we live. Our goal should be to create a healthy lifestyle in which we eat and maintain physical activities so that our body parts keep functioning well, including our brains. Part of this goal should be including more positives in our lives by deleting self-defeating terms such as *diet*.

So I have stopped using the word *diet*. I have wasted a good part of my life agonizing, punishing myself, and ultimately crying over this word. I have wasted precious time with friends, family, and my husband, whining about this subject over and over and over again. I refuse to give one more precious moment to this vile word. I have stopped talking to others about my weight, and I have stopped using the word *diet*.

No more ranting and raving over this subject. I have hyperventilated about this topic so often while on my nightly walk with my husband that I'm sure he feared I would give myself a heart attack by stressing so much about why I just couldn't lose the weight once and for all. Our walks ceased being quiet, relaxing time together. I continued to rant and rave about knowing what to do about losing weight and even how great I'd feel accomplishing it. I am a strong-willed person, but, ultimately, I couldn't do it. Even my husband was perplexed as to why I couldn't lose the excess weight. This nonstop obsessing was extremely unhealthy for both of us, yet I couldn't stop.

This would mean defeat, and I would never accept that I was going to be this size or even bigger for the rest of my life.

With all my references to the devil, I want to believe that an angel finally stepped in to guide me. Somehow, I just stopped. I stopped all the negative thoughts and the mindless ranting and raving. I became calm, and I tried a new approach.

My new philosophy is to be positive regarding my health. Instead of using the word diet, I now use a few phrases that are fun and sassy yet still speak the truth. The first phrase I chose was *big butt removal*. This obviously defines my first problem area. I chose to add laughter to my life every day, so why not choose a comical phrase for my new perspective on losing weight? A funnier version of *big butt removal* is *big kitako removal*, with *kitako* being *butt* in Swahili. Who knew?

Another phrase I use is *gimme skinny*. This phrase refers to my legs only. My goal is not to be a twig but to gain that free feeling when you walk and your thighs don't slap each other.

Now I giggle to myself when I think of my personal goals. Remember that previous chapter on laughter? It works. I have applied laughter to this area of my life and will use this positive energy to help me on my big kitako removal journey.

Just eliminating the despicable word *diet* from my life has made me breathe slower. I have freed myself from a lifetime of obsessing over dieting and have begun a new lifestyle. I laugh more when gently reminding myself of my goals and have honestly become a happier person. You can, too.

Try it! Choose a new word or phrase for yourself, something that will make you smile, laugh, whatever it takes to give you a more positive outlook on weight loss.

Feel free to improvise your own term. Be creative—after all this is *your* plan!

Some suggestions:

Earth Goddess Plan	Operation Bikini Babe
Nature's Spirit Program	Hot Momma Plan
Feeling Groovy Program	Cowgirl Plan*

Go to the website: www.sassy-gal.com for more ideas, and tell me yours!

---

*Cowgirl Plan: don't all gals wish they could wear those skinny jeans tucked into a fabulous pair of cowgirl boots and yell, "Yippee, cay yea!" Go for this one.

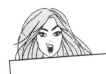

17

Put Yourself First

My idea of family means everyone participates. How could we experience the happiness of being part of a family if the work and pleasure parts were unevenly distributed? We all have titles, but we each share most of the same responsibilities. Each family member helps prepare meals, clean the house, do yard chores, and take care of the dog.

It is my responsibility to teach my kids independence and to guide them along in this endeavor. I am their parent, not their servant. When I became a mother, I looked at this as if I were given another title. I did not lose my previous title of individual. I certainly have more responsibilities, but I must also take care of myself by putting myself first every now and then. I can't wait until every family problem is solved before it's my turn. We all know my turn would never come.

Look at this from your family's perspective: They will appreciate you sacrificing for them, but they will also feel sorry for you if you aren't strong enough to take care of yourself, too. If you are over-weight, they may not only feel sorry for you but also be embarrassed for you or resent you. There is a time when you may be sacrificing too much for your family's sake. You might be the perfect loving parent, but if you can't control your own weight you may look like a loser in your child's eyes. Don't help your family move forward while leaving yourself behind.

When your children are off on their own, will they look back at their childhood with feelings of respect or disappointment toward you as their parent? Take care of yourself first, for everyone's sake.

18

We Need to Have the "Joy of . . ." Talk

Yes, we need to have the "Joy" talk. Why? Because you don't find joy in overeating!

Like many Americans, I find what I believe to be joy through most food at any time. For me, joy would be a nonstop, calorie-free smorgasbord. I think about food constantly, including in my dreams. While I'm eating breakfast I think about lunch, during lunch I think about what is for dinner, and on and on. I love food and I obsess about it. I am embarrassed that I am over 50 years old and am admitting that food is a major goal in my life. I've never really put it into perspective before, but the truth is that I have placed too much emphasis on food.

I am sure I am not alone when I disclose the fact that food is an integral part of our family trips. Each trip requires a specific dessert. We bring berry pie to the lake, chocolate cupcakes to the cabin, and brownies to the ocean, where we add ice cream. It's been the same desserts for years. Heaven help me if I change any of them. My kids associate the desserts with each trip, as they always remind me to make a specific dessert to take with us, as if the desserts were part of our personal belongings. It seems as if our joy depends on which eating event we're attending next.

So how do we rewire our brains? More important, should we? We shouldn't. Food will always be part of our celebrations. We'd be fools to think otherwise. And besides, if pie and chocolate and ice cream are our only vices, that's not so bad.

So I've decided to try to make eating a "subjoy." In other words, I will find other joyous moments to renew my spirit that won't make me depend so much on food. I need a daily ritual all to myself that I can look forward to and that will bring me contentment.

I didn't have to think too long about this one. My family enjoys being outdoors. My parents gave me the greatest gift: family time that included travel adventures. We traveled by car and camped at all of our destinations either in tents, trailers, or cabins. We hiked, rode bikes, swam, and cooked over campfires. My parents gave me the pure, simple joy of being outdoors, feeling free and adventurous. We had the perfect balance of exercise and caloric intake.

My favorite memory is when my dad would get home from work in the late afternoon in the summer. He would yell to my mom to get our bathing suits while he packed the portable grill, because we were headed for the lake, a short 30 minutes away. I can still *feel* those memories. Late afternoon summer days at the lake can be incredible. Somehow the wind dies down, the water is calm and warmed by the full day of sun, and the sun is still warm but doesn't scorch you. After a nice swim in the fresh water, you can actually sunbathe without scrunching your eyes closed and you can totally relax. The sand on the beach is comforting because it is warm rather than unbearably hot. The crowds are long gone and you have the entire area to yourself. Add the smell and taste of grilled hot dogs, and everyone is happy. It's simple yet wonderful. A moment of pure joy. This simple activity at this special spot is what truly rejuvenates me.

Whether I can make it to the beach or not, my goal will be to do something I enjoy in the latter part of the day. Sunny afternoons will be my new joy, whether I swim or just sit barefoot in my comfy chair by the window while I work. Food will now be my subjoy.

This is about how you really want to live your life. I'm talking about the down-to-earth, simple joys, not the fantasy life you imagine and never achieve. Close your eyes if you have to. Find what really feeds your spirit and can be incorporated daily into your life and routines. Choose something that won't change as you age, move, or end because friendships change. This means choosing something that you have control over.

Now that you've chosen your joyous daily ritual, the joy = food paradigm will shift to joy = simple daily ritual.

Only on special occasions should food be considered part of the attraction. You should have a special reason to overindulge, such as weddings, birthdays, and celebration dinners. These are not everyday events, and the quality of food must be worth the temptation. Distinguish what foods are worth the calories. If the food doesn't make you go mmm, then leave it. Is that cake served at the office birthday party really worth the extra calories, or are you just eating that generic stuff because it is free and creates a good excuse to stop working?

Now I understand why my family won't let me change our trip desserts. They truly are delicious and are a part of our family celebrations. Besides, you absolutely can't go through life without really good chocolate and a fabulous chocolate cake recipe (see the next page).

Sassy Gal Chocolate Cake

½ cup Dutch-processed cocoa
  powder
1 cup water
2 cups cake flour
2 cups sugar
1 teaspoon salt
1½ teaspoons baking soda
1 cup buttermilk
¾ cup vegetable oil
2 large eggs, beaten lightly
1 teaspoon vanilla

Frosting:
½ pound unsalted butter
1 ounce bittersweet chocolate
1 ounce semisweet chocolate
3 ounces unsweetened
  chocolate
1 to 2 ounces German sweet
  chocolate
1 teaspoon vanilla
1 pound confectioners' sugar
¼ to ⅓ cup sour cream

1. Preheat oven to 350 degrees. Grease and flour cake pans.
2. In a saucepan set over medium heat, combine the water and cocoa powder. Whisk the mixture until smooth and let cool.
3. In a bowl, sift the flour, sugar, salt, and baking soda. In another bowl, whisk together the buttermilk, vegetable oil, eggs, and vanilla.
4. Add the buttermilk mixture to the flour, stirring until combined. Stir in the cocoa powder mixture. Transfer the batter to the prepared pans and bake for 30 to 35 minutes or until a cake tester inserted in the center comes out clean. Transfer to a rack to cool completely.

To make the frosting:
1. In a microwave, melt the butter and chocolates (1–2 minutes), stirring occasionally. Add vanilla and let cool. Using a hand mixer, add the sugar and sour cream, a little at a time. If necessary, chill until firm enough to spread.
2. Frost cake and enjoy!

19

One Simple Change Equals a Life-Changing Moment

Nutritionists and doctors, including Dr. Mehmet Oz, suggest that you always eat the same breakfast.

When I first heard this statement, I rolled my eyes. After I heard the explanation, my eyes became focused because it made sense. And it was literally life changing.

We have all heard the advice: eat a nutritious breakfast because it is the most important meal of the day. That's a lot of pressure to face so early in the day, not to mention that someone is telling you what to do as soon as you wake up. But it sure would be nice to not have to think about one meal a day. Lunch and dinner are such challenges themselves.

I tried it. The key is finding breakfast foods that are beneficial, containing fiber and no excess amounts of sugar or preservatives. You know the drill: most prepackaged breakfast foods are not the answer here.

So I cruised the supermarket breakfast aisle, looking at cereals. Yuck. I hate most cereals. And eat them every day? I needed to be creative here. I bought several boxes of high-fiber, high-nutrient cereals with low sugar content, and I mixed them together. I made individual servings, adding dried fruits, and then taste-tested. Not bad.

Dutch Baby

3 golden delicious apples, peeled and cut into ¼-inch wedges
½ cup dried cherries
2 tablespoons butter
6 tablespoons sugar
½ teaspoon almond extract
½ cup apple juice or apple cider
⅓ cup all-purpose flour
⅓ cup whole wheat flour
1 cup skim milk
¼ teaspoon salt
3 large eggs, lightly beaten
1 tablespoon powdered sugar

1. Preheat oven to 425 degrees.
2. Melt 1 tablespoon butter in a 10-inch cast-iron or oven-proof skillet over medium-high heat. Add the apples, cherries, 3 tablespoons of the sugar, and the almond extract, and cook until the apples are tender, about 10 minutes. Add the apple juice, and cook 1 to 2 more minutes until liquid is slightly thickened. Transfer to a separate dish.
3. In a separate bowl, whisk the milk, 3 tablespoons of sugar, salt, and eggs. Add flours and whisk until well blended.
4. Melt 1 tablespoon of butter in the 10-inch cast-iron skillet. Pour the batter into the skillet, and bake until puffy and golden, 18 to 22 minutes. Add apples and cherries on top, sprinkle with powdered sugar, and serve.

I could do this. Then I added toasted almonds. Yum. I now eat this cereal mixture Monday through Friday, and I have heartier breakfasts with my family on the weekends. We have omelets, frittatas, and Dutch babies. These weekend breakfasts are loaded with vegetables, salmon, and fruit, so we are pleased with our choices. By the way, if you have never tried a Dutch baby pancake, try the one on the previous page.

For a little variety during the week, I might have oatmeal (remember how comforting that can be) or a pumpkin muffin. The result? Success. I no longer stress about breakfast. Forget about last night's leftover pizza. I will look forward to that for lunch. And forget about cooking. I just grab my cereal packet, add almond milk, coconut milk or a soy drink, and I am done. It's as easy as that.

This was life changing for me. Just look at the *permanent* benefits of this one simple change:

- No more daily morning decisions; my mornings are calm and pleasurable without ugly food-choice episodes.
- I have a super-charged breakfast. I avoid excess sugars, fats, and preservatives.
- Fiber creates "righteous" poop.
- It stops me from giving in to nighttime food commercials. Marketers, I now control you!
- I avoid tons of worthless calories.

Most important, I have gained some control in my life! My new body is very happy. Thank you, nutritionists and Dr. Oz.

Breakfast Ideas

Please note that the following recipes emphasize fiber content. These recipes were created using minimal amounts of sugars and oils in an effort to maintain flavor. Feel free to adjust these amounts to your personal taste preferences and needs.

Nutty Harvest Grain Pancakes

¾ cup oats
¼ cup slivered almonds
¼ cup pecans
¾ cup whole wheat flour
⅓ cup all-purpose flour
2 teaspoons baking soda
1 teaspoon baking powder
½ teaspoon salt

1¼ cups buttermilk
⅓ cup whole milk
¼ cup vegetable oil
2 eggs
¼ cup sugar
½ cup chopped walnuts (or pecans)

1. Grind the oats, almonds, and ¼ cup walnuts or pecans in a food processor or blender until fine.
2. Combine with whole wheat flour, all-purpose flour, baking soda, baking powder, and salt in a large bowl.
3. In another bowl combine buttermilk, milk, oil, eggs, and sugar with electric mixer until smooth.
4. Combine all, adding ½ cup chopped walnuts or pecans, and mix well by hand.
5. Ladle batter onto lightly oiled, medium-hot skillet and cook 1 to 3 minutes per side. Makes 12 pancakes.

Pumpkin Muffins

¾ cup whole wheat flour
½ cup all-purpose flour
½ cup sugar
½ teaspoon cinnamon
½ teaspoon nutmeg
½ teaspoon pumpkin pie spice
½ teaspoon ground cloves
½ teaspoon salt

1 teaspoon baking powder
½ teaspoon baking soda
½ cup applesauce
¼ cup vegetable oil
1 cup pumpkin (canned)
1 egg
½ cup raisins
½ cup pecans

1. Preheat the oven to 350 degrees. Lightly grease muffin pan.
2. Combine dry ingredients in large bowl. Combine wet ingredients in separate bowl. Mix all together, adding raisins and pecans. Bake for 18–25 minutes. Makes 12 muffins. These muffins freeze beautifully.

Creamy Fruit Delight

2 cups vanilla Greek yogurt (or
   non-fat vanilla yogurt)
2 tablespoons honey
2 bananas, peeled and cut into
   slices

1 cup fresh or frozen blueberries*
1 cup granola

Mix together the yogurt and honey (this makes the dish creamier, almost like a dessert). Add the bananas and blueberries. Spoon into dishes or tall glasses. Sprinkle granola on top. Serves 4.

*Note: Sweet black cherries, peaches, strawberries, raspberries, or a mixture of fruits will also taste great.

20

One Giant Baby Step (Gulp Water)

I am one of those individuals who hate the taste of water. I certainly know the importance of water for our bodies, but I despise drinking it. Current theories on how foods actually give us a major source of our daily water needs is comforting, but I know that I must supplement my water intake to ensure that I do not become dehydrated. Since I refuse to drink those sugary flavored waters or artificially sweetened water, what am I and others like me to do?

Gulp it down.

You heard me. Instead of torturing yourself throughout the day taking small sips of water, take your entire glass and gulp it down. Just get it over with. I watched someone do this after a gym workout. The person was literally chugging down the entire contents of a water bottle. It dawned on me that most people drink a lot of water quickly during their workouts and immediately after. They do it to quickly rehydrate themselves. Why shouldn't I do the same? Every morning, I now chug a glass of water. I chug it at a pace that avoids choking, of course. Then I repeat this later in the day.

This is what I mean when I talk about one small change making a significant permanent difference. I have found a way to add more water to my body, painlessly.

21

Go Green!

$\mathcal{S}$ome of you read books on diet, exercise, and nutrition with good intentions but become immediately overwhelmed after reading them. For you, I suggest baby steps that will dramatically change your life in other ways first. The following may help you become stronger by removing chemicals from your home, helping you feed your soul, and helping you find inner peace through simple joys. Maybe then you can go back to your personal body improvement plan.

All you have to do is go green: include nature in your life.

Detox Your House

Nature can be very generous. Not only does it provide greens to feed our bodies with but it also provides greens to keep our lungs healthy. Green plants detoxify the air for us, so add them to your indoor spaces. I did some research on this topic to see which chemicals were harmful and which plants could remove them from the air. Three common hazardous chemicals are:

- **Benzene:** Used in the manufacture of plastics, detergents, pharmaceuticals, and dyes. Health risks include cancer, leukemia, drowsiness, dizziness, unconsciousness, and death.
- **Formaldehyde:** Found in virtually all indoor environments. Major sources include particle-board or pressed-wood furniture, carpeting, grocery bags, waxed paper, facial tissue, paper towels, and many household cleaning products. Health risks include nasal and lung cancer, possibly brain cancer and leukemia, eczema, respiratory difficulty, and death.
- **Trichloroethylene:** Found in printing inks, paints, lacquers, varnishes and adhesives, and spot removers. Health risks include headaches; lung irritation; dizziness; poor coordination; concentration difficulties; unconsciousness; nerve, kidney, and liver damage; and death.

NASA has done extensive research on green plants' air-purifying effects in developing life-support systems for space stations. Its research has shown that many common house plants can clean the air of toxic gases. The top 10 air-purifying plants according to NASA are:

1. Areca palm
2. Lady palm
3. Bamboo palm
4. Rubber plant (caution: plant leaves are toxic to humans and pets)
5. Dracaena
6. English ivy
7. Dwarf date palm

8. Ficus alii
9. Boston fern
10. Peace lily

Note: Not all plants are good indoor air cleaners. Many house plants can actually be toxic themselves. Research a plant before bringing it into your home.

Grow Your Own Garden

At least once in your lifetime, grow something. Let nature feed your soul. Experience firsthand the pure joy of watching something grow that you planted with your own two hands. I don't care how rich you are or how manicured your nails are. Get outside and plant. Be able to proclaim before you die that you got your hands dirty and actually gardened. It's as easy as this:

1. Buy seeds or plants from the store.
2. Spend 10 minutes digging a hole, adding nutrients, and planting seeds or plants.
3. Spend 5 minutes putting a small fence or netting around plants.
4. Water regularly.
5. Watch your garden grow.
6. Smirk. You actually did it, Farmer Brown!

I guarantee that you will get unbelievable personal satisfaction from this. The moment you pick your first tomato, strawberry, pumpkin, or flower will be joyous. Not corny or not old-fashioned, but joyous.

Connect with Nature

Take advantage of nature's beauty and its ability to remove stress from your life. Adding peacefulness to your life can be as simple as adding an Adirondack chair to your backyard or that hammock that you've been talking about. Send the kids outside with a blanket for their own picnic. Add a garden table and chairs where you could enjoy an outdoor meal or glass of wine. How about adding a new tree to your yard so you can watch it blossom or watch its leaves change colors? I particularly enjoy watching birds at a bird feeder. I have one directly outside my kitchen window, and I feel myself relax every time I see or hear those sweet birds. Add plants that will attract butterflies and hummingbirds to your yard. This is cheap and easy, and it yields wonderful results. City dwellers can create their own indoor garden space. A plant next to a chair will bring the outdoors in.

If this green stuff is new to you, go to any garden center during the springtime and watch others as they eagerly select their plants and garden supplies. It is a happy place. I have never seen an angry gardener or one who uses profanity while gardening. They may talk or sing to themselves, yes, but not cuss. This is definitely a good thing. If you aren't connecting with nature in some way, you have missed the point of being on this planet. Nature is peaceful, calming, and joyous.

TROUBLESHOOTING

DISPLAY	SITUATION	SOLUTION/EXPLANATION
No Wt. Displayed	No Weight Displayed	Check if scale has been powered up please refer to the "Preparation" Section.
"LO"	Batteries are running low	Replace batteries as a simultaneous set.
"O-LD"	Overload warning	Remove the weight immediately.
"Err"	Instability error	Step off the scale and wait for scale to switch off automatically. Step on scale to repeat the measurement process remain still while the scale is processing. Scale must be on flat, level, hard surface.
"Err"	Estimated body fat percentage is beyond the technical limit	Moistening your feet may help improve the surface contact.
"Err"	Contact error	Please make sure you are standing still on the scale and making maximum contact between your feet and the metal contacts. You may need to moisten your feet to improve the surface contact.
Numeric	Weight is not measuring properly	Check to be sure scale is set to the desired measurement (lb,kg,st)
Blank	Not functioning	Check to be sure batteries are installed correctly.

If problems persist after troubleshooting remove the batteries, wait one minute, and replace.

Why do I get a different reading when I use a different brand of body fat scale? Different body fat scales take estimations around different parts of the body and use different mathematical algorithms to estimate the percentage of body fat. The best advice is to not make comparisons from one device to another, but to use the same device each time to monitor any change.

ELECTRONIC SCALE FG9301 ONE YEAR LIMITED WARRANTY
DO NOT RETURN THIS PRODUCT TO THE STORE

BIGWALL warrants that during the first year from the original date of purchase, this product will be free from defects in material and workmanship. Bigwall, at its discretion, will repair or replace this product or any component of this product found to be defective during the warranty period. This is a one-time replacement warranty. If the product is no longer available, Bigwall will replace the unit with a similar model of equal or greater value. This warranty is not transferable. Proof of purchase is REQUIRED in order to obtain warranty assistance.

This warranty does NOT cover:
• Negligent use or misuse of the product.
• Damages as the result of not using product in accordance with provided instructions.
• Water damage
• Additional or extended warranties offered by retailers.
• Disassembly or repair by anyone other than an authorized Bigwall service center Products used in a commercial setting.
• Floor display or 'as-is' models.
• Damage caused by acts of nature such as hurricane, tornado, fire, etc.
• Incidental or consequential damages caused by breach of any expressed, implied or Any performance issues that fall
  outside of the 1 year warranty.

Note: Some states do not allow the exclusion or limitation of incidental or consequential damages. This limitation or exclusion may not apply to you.

If you have any questions about this product or its warranty, please call customer service at toll-free **1-877-365-6274.**

FCC STATEMENT

PLEASE NOTE THAT CHANGES OR MODIFICATIONS NOT EXPRESSLY APPROVED BY THE PARTY RESPONSIBLE FOR COMPLIANCE COULD VOID THE USER'S AUTHORITY TO OPERATE THE EQUIPMENT.

POTENTIAL FOR RADIO/TELEVISION INTERFERENCE

This product has been tested and found to comply with the limits for a Class B digital device, pursuant to part 15 of the FCC rules. These limits are designed to provide reasonable protection against harmful interference in a residential installation.

The product generates, uses, and can radiate radio frequency energy and, if not installed and used accordance with the instructions, may cause harmful interference to radio communications.

However, there is no guarantee that the interference will not occur in a particular installation. If the product does cause harmful interference to radio or television reception, which can be determined by turning the product on or off, the user is encouraged to try to correct the interference by one or more of the following measures:

a) Reorient or relocate the receiving antenna;
b) Increase the separation between the product and the receiver;
c) Consult an experienced radio/TV technician for help.

Changes or modifications not expressly approved by the party responsible for compliance could void the user's authority to operate the equipment.

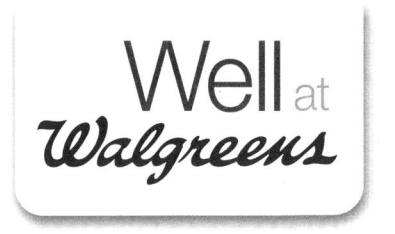

Digital Glass Scale
with body analysis features

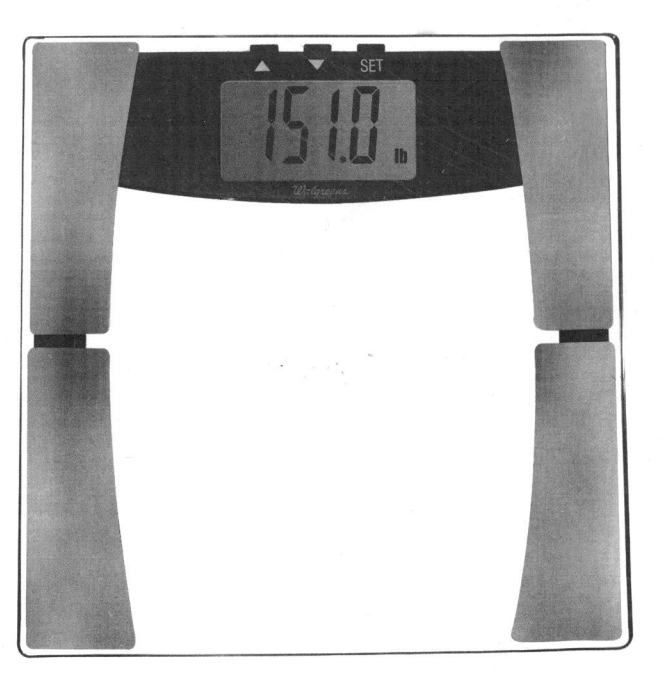

USER MANUAL

BE SURE TO SAVE THESE INSTRUCTIONS ALONG WITH YOUR RECEIPT

...s to familiarize yourself with the features and operations before programming the scale.

...not recommended for persons with an electronic implant (heart pacemaker).

...late body fat unless you are barefoot.
...at estimate, do not bend your knees, keep your legs/thighs apart and straight when standing on the scale.
...s not recommended for use by pregnant women, persons with fever, swollen legs or other edemas, as well as a ...lrated or dehydrated.
...nay be slightly higher or lower for children under 16, persons with diabetes and other health conditions.
...approximately 5% more body fat than men.

...AAA batteries (included). Open the battery cover on the back of the scale unit and insert the batteries. Be sure the ...correct for the scale to function properly. If you do not intend to use this unit for prolonged periods of time, it is ...batteries before storing.

...ion
...a flat and hard floor surface. Do not use on carpets or uneven surfaces. DO NOT place near a bathtub or shower.

...ment
...to pounds, press firmly on the platform to turn the scale on. Press [set] to toggle between pounds (lb), kilogram (kg) ...easurement. Allow the scale to turn off. The scale is set to function in the unit last displayed.

...e platform to turn on the scale, the display shows 0.0lb. The scale is ready for use.

...rams kg, Stones st or pounds lb)
Centimeters

Feet and Inches

...CTION
...o get your weight measurement, simply use the Instant On or Tap On methods below

...Tap the center of the platform. Step away from scale and wait for 0.0 to appear. Step on scale.
...s - Step on scale

...position your feet so that your weight is distributed evenly over the scale platform. Stand still while the scale ...The LCD will display your weight within a few seconds. Stand still while reading is displayed.

BODY FAT AND TOTAL BODY WATER ESTIMATING OPERATION

1. Press the [SET] key to turn on.
2. **Set memory** - Press the [▲] or [▼] key to select a memory location (1-12 user). Press [SET] to confirm.
3. **Select unit of measurement** - Your scale is set to first display in pounds (lb). Press [SET] to select. Or press the [▲] or [▼] key to toggle between lb (pound), kg(kilograms) and st (stone). Press [SET] to confirm the displayed unit of measurement.
4. **Select gender** - Press the [▲] or [▼] key to toggle between the male and female icons. Press [SET] to confirm gender.
5. **Set age** - Press the [▲] or [▼] key to adjust the age. Press [SET] to confirm.
6. **Set height** - Press the [▲] or [▼] key to adjust the height. Press [SET] to confirm.
7. **Set normal or athlete mode** - Press the [▲] or [▼] key to toggle between normal (no icon) and athlete mode. Press [SET] to confirm all settings. **NOTE:** Athlete mode is only available for those 18-70 years of age. For those ages 17 or under and 71 or over. This step is automatically by-passed.
8. All personal information stored to memory will be displayed. The scale will show " 0.0 " after a few seconds. Your personal information is saved in memory. **NOTE:** You may step on the scale for a reading with bare feet when "0.0 " appears on the screen. When the scale turns off your personal memory is saved in memory.
9. Repeat steps 1-8 to set other pre-programmed user numbers.

TO RECALL SETTINGS FROM MEMORY FOR BODY FAT AND TOTAL BODY WATER ESTIMATION

You must have bare feet for estimation results. Remove your shoes and socks before proceeding. Clean, slightly moist feet will provide the best results. Position your feet for maximum contact with the metal surfaces on the scale platform.

1. Press the [SET] key to turn the scale on.
2. Press the [▲] or [▼] key to toggle between memory locations (1-12). The screen will show the previous personal data screens, then "0.0".
3. When "0.0" appears on the screen, step on the scale with bare feet, positioning your feet evenly on the scale platform with maximum contact with the metal electrodes.
4. Stand still while the scale measures your weight and estimates your body composition.
5. Your weight, body fat %, total body water %, BMI, muscle mass, bone mass and daily calorie estimates/ basal metabolic rate (Kcal/BMR) are displayed.

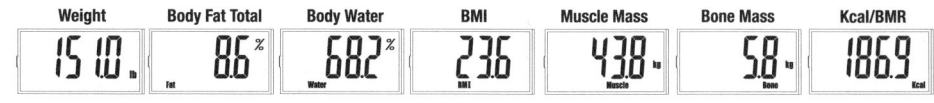

Weight	Body Fat Total	Body Water	BMI	Muscle Mass	Bone Mass	Kcal/BMR
151.0 lb	8.6 % Fat	68.2 % Water	23.6 BMI	43.8 kg Muscle	5.8 kg Bone	186.9 Kcal

6. The results are repeated, and then the scale will turn off automatically.

REVIEW ANALYSIS DATA

1. Press the [SET] key to turn the scale on. Then the screen display the user number, wait for a few seconds, until the screen display "0.0".
2. If you want to review the last analysis data, press the [▲] key, then the user number show on the screen. Press the [▲] or [▼] key to choose your memory location number (1-12).
3. Press the [SET] key to confirm your number, then the analysis data will be displayed one by one.

PRODUCT SPECIFICATIONS

1. Capacity: 180kg/400lb/28st
2. Graduation: 0.1kg/0.2lb/1st (0.2lb when the weight is less than 20st, 1lb when the weight is 20st or over)
3. Body fat graduation: 0.1%
4. Body water graduation: 0.1%
5. Bone mass graduation: 0.1kg/0.1lb
6. Muscle mass graduation: 0.1kg/0.1lb
7. Age range from 6 to 100 years
8. Height range from 2'8" to 7'2" (80 to 220 cm)
9. Body fat range: 5 to 65%
10. Total body water range: 20 to 80%
11. Operates with 2 AAA batteries (included)

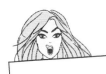

22

Obliterate the Word Exercise from Your Vocabulary

*M*ost of us hate to exercise, hate the thought of exercising, even hate the word *exercise*. And no one wants to be told to exercise.

We know exercise is essential, but we don't want to do it. The word *exercise* has become synonymous with sweat-inducing hard labor and is a life sentence, with no possibility of parole.

The word has such a negative meaning that I bet it's one of the top 10 most disliked words in English. Thousands of web pages are devoted to the excuses people give to not have to exercise. People will just tune out when confronted with this word.

The number-one reason for not exercising is not having time to exercise. This excuse is just plain ridiculous. Grow up. Especially someone my age should feel utterly foolish if she ever says this and, worse yet, believes it. While we are at it, let's stop allowing people to use this excuse. From now on, if you hear people say that they have no time for exercise, feel free to tell them to shut up. We all know that what they are really saying is that they choose to not exercise. Let's not give anyone permission ever again to use this flimsy excuse.

The more we hate the word *exercise*, the more we will gloss over it and ignore it. Fitness experts intensify our hatred for the word by portraying exercise as meaningless unless we do cardio *and* calisthenics *and* strength training *and* flexibility routines. This is unrealistic for most of us. Thus, the word *exercise* can actually immobilize you because the task seems so daunting and impossible. No wonder we hate this word. Besides, who should we listen to? Which doctors? Which fitness experts? Forget about the no-pain, no-gain attitude. It's not for me.

You have to be fit for survival. You need to keep your body parts in good working order, but you don't have to be king of the jungle. If you enjoy exercising until exhaustion, good for you! Feel free to put down this wimpy book and give me 50!

As you did for diet, create your own word for exercise. Health experts have been trying to do this for decades, using *fitness training, body shaping, healthy lifestyle,* and *body sculpting,* to name just a few. None of these phrases work for me. These words have less negative meanings than *exercise,* but they are still derogatory. *Body shaping* tells me that I'd better not show my body in public because the fat on my outer thighs slaps people as I go by. *Body sculpting?* Please. If I could sculpt the fat off my butt and redirect it to where it belongs, I'd be teaching the Barbie Body Workout. And don't get me started on the *healthy lifestyle* gimmick. I resent this phrase. To imply that I am unhealthy because I am 10 pounds overweight, don't jog five miles a day, and don't grow my own organic food is preposterous. Unhealthy for whom? I am doing the best I can with my limitations as an earthling and with all the minefields that are in my path.

I needed something more personal, more meaningful, to my life. I thought about how daily exercise affected me and how much I needed. If you think about it, your body will tell you when you need to move. Just like a child who wiggles when restrained, your body craves to move. When you've been sitting too long, your butt actually becomes numb. Think of those long car rides when you keep shifting positions or when you watch TV too long. You can feel your legs getting cramps or starting to fall asleep. Your brain even slows down. I start feeling antsy and have to move around.

This is the main reason why I disliked so many nine-to-five jobs. My body and mind did not like others telling me how long I had to stay chained to my desk and chair. My goal was never to achieve that big corner office and big comfy chair but to gain my freedom from it.

My body craves to be free, and I replaced exercise with *free spirit time*. To me, this phrase encompasses all forms of body movement, including dancing wildly to music and chasing my dog around the house. She, too, needs exercise, and she loves to be chased. I found that the more I swung my arms wildly at her, yelled using crazy voices, or stomped loudly with my feet while on pursuit, the more she loved it. She gets as bored as I do playing fetch with the same old toys. Instead, she will grab an item in the house, such as a placemat from the table, and stand in front of me with it, knowing that I will chase her to retrieve it. As you can imagine, this is not only a way for the dog and me to move our old bones, but it is also an incredible way to release stress. I just hope the neighbors understand that a crazy lady doesn't live next door to them!

Another idea is an elliptical machine. This piece of equipment is brilliant. You can glide on it or move like a maniac. It's easy and effective. No bones pounding the pavement for miles in inclement weather. I can let my body move freely for as long or little as I need. I select my music, and my free spirit time is over before I know it. I can even close my eyes while using it.

I also realized that I need freedom from the indoors. I need to physically leave my house every day to be with people and especially to enjoy the outdoors. So I walk with my husband. It has become a time to unwind and relax, just wandering in nature. (I am, of course, no longer talking or obsessing about my weight.)

My favorite is swimming. Doing a slow breaststroke or sidestroke or even floating can be the most relaxing thing. I want my tombstone to read "Lake's Open!"

My body told me what I needed. I need to be a free spirit, so this is what I will call my exercise time.

Exercise is necessary for the body and mind, but don't let the word *exercise* hold you back. Oprah wrote in her February 2010 *O, The Oprah Magazine,* that she stopped calling it *exercise.* She looks at it as honoring the body, which carries life and is life itself. Let go of the word *exercise.* Find your own word and meaning, and take control of your physical wellbeing. I made a brand-new start in my life and you can too.

Some suggestions:

Find your mojo   Get your groove on

Move old bones	Spread your wings
Zoezi*	

Go to the website: www.sassy-gal.com for more ideas and to tell me yours!

Zoezi is *exercise* in Swahili.

23

Vitamins and Minerals: Why Foods Are Good for You

Sure, we know that we need vitamins and minerals. We know foods that contain them are "good for you." But it has been a really long time since I've studied basic nutrition. How do our individual body parts really use nutrition to function? It was time for a review. I went to the USDA website (www.choosemyplate.gov) to review food basics. I reviewed the charts and data and reeducated myself on how amazing and complex the human body is. I had forgotten that the human body is quite the chemistry set and was fascinated by the fact that magnesium is needed for more than 300 biochemical reactions in the body. In living cells, chemical reactions take place that help sustain life and allow cells to grow. I guess there are no true human couch potatoes.

The USDA website gives detailed information on every food group, including the nutrients each provides and the health benefits of each.

It is important to note that this is only one source of information. You may choose to research food nutrition as much as your healthy heart desires.

It seems that what most experts in the health field have been preaching to us makes sense. Eating a variety of foods is the key. (Experts prefer to use the term *well-balanced diet*.) Even if the experts disagree on the specifics of each, I can protect myself by eating a variety of these everyday foods, with a little of the junk food I crave, as long as I keep a commonsense attitude about it.

I do have to admit, though, that I will not be including beef or chicken livers, cod liver oil, or oysters to my plates, even if these are super-foods. Maybe the food industry could develop a product from a combination of these items to create the ultimate super-food patty. On second thought. . . .

24

Become a Vegevore

Let's get serious about fats. Go ahead, pinch a fat area of your body (your thigh for example) and hold onto it. Hold it, squeeze it, and squish it all around while you ponder where the hell it came from. What did you gain your excess fat from? The way the body makes fat is actually an extremely complex process involving hundreds of different chemical reactions and dozens of nutrients. Determining exactly how you got the excess fat you're now pondering over may take a chemist to analyze, but I suspect you already have a good idea as to how it got there. I certainly do. I know that my excess fat wasn't a result of eating too much fruit and vegetables. I was overindulging in other things, especially the unhealthy stuff.

Most Westerners are omnivores. We feed on both animals and plants, eating all kinds of foods indiscriminately. We know the solution to ridding our bodies of excess fat is to decrease our intake of fats and increase our intake of fruits, vegetables, and whole grains, incorporating more of a vegetarian diet. The new MyPlate guideline created by the USDA to replace the former Food Pyramid supports this.

MyPlate guidelines recommend that at least half of your meal should consist of fruits and vegetables, and the other half consist of grains (preferably whole grains) and protein. The emphasis is definitely on getting people to eat more fruits, vegetables, and whole grains.

The best-selling book *The China Study* by T. Colin Campbell, PhD, and Thomas M. Campbell II focuses on Dr. Campbell's years of nutrition research on the multiple health benefits of consuming a plant-based diet. The evidence is compelling. Such diseases as heart disease, cancer, diabetes, arthritis, and other chronic diseases can be minimized by consuming a low-fat, plant-based diet. According to the research, plant-based foods contain no cholesterol and high amounts of fiber, while animal products contain cholesterol and no fiber. *The China Study* not only recommends eating a plant-based diet but also eliminating all animal products, including milk, cheese, and eggs.

According to Dr. Campbell, we will live healthier lives and lose weight if we eat a low-fat, low–animal-protein diet high in complex carbohydrates from fruits and vegetables.

Our minds and bodies want us to eat better so that we can perform better. But to follow Dr. Campbell's recommendations, we are once again asked to drastically change our current eating habits overnight. We are not only asked to give up our omnivore way of eating but told to go straight to veganism, which completely omits all animal products, including milk, cheese, and eggs. This is an impossible task for most of us. Many of us can't even get to the vegetarian stage, which allows some animal products (e.g., dairy).

If this eating regimen seems too drastic, there may be a way we can take a very large baby step first. Let's explore a new category. Let's strive first to be vegevores.

In 2005 a few hundred people in Portland, Oregon, began celebrating an annual VegFest, calling themselves vegevores. The festival is meant to attract people who want to share their passion for vegetables. The vegevores stress that their mantra is their love of vegetables rather than hatred of meat. Their mission is to have vegetables occupy most of the plate, adding meat for flavor only. They are not opposed to eating meat; they just choose to emphasize vegetables. The annual Portland VegFest continues today, and other vegevores around the country are starting their own groups to encourage this type of eating.

By becoming vegevores, we will strive to increase our consumption of fruits and vegetables while decreasing our consumption of meat and animal products. Notice that the emphasis is on fruits and vegetables, but we are allowed minimum amounts of animal products. This differs from omnivores, for whom the proportion of animals to plants is not specified. We won't eliminate animal products; we will just limit them as best we can.

We can do this by serving smaller portions of meat, fowl, and seafood. We can also add more vegetarian meals. Vegetables have numerous advantages and are considered superstars by nutritionists. Vegetables are high-fiber, high-water complex carbohydrates, which help keep people's weight under control. They also contain vitamins and minerals while being low in calories and fat. Vegetables also contain potent antioxidants, which may help protect against cellular damage.

Food Consumption Categories

Omnivore: eats animals and plants indiscriminately

Vegevore: eats mostly plants and small amounts of animal and animal products (e.g., dairy)

Vegetarian: eats plants and animal products, but not animal flesh
Vegan: eats plants only

Here are some suggestions for becoming a vegevore:

- Decrease the amounts of meats, fowl, and fish you eat by serving smaller pieces. Instead of serving a whole piece of beef or chicken, serve slices or strips.
- Eat no-fat or low-fat cheese, and use shredded cheese to decrease the serving size. Experiment with spicy cheeses such as pepper jack cheese to maximize flavor while using smaller amounts.
- Try soy, coconut, and almond milk. They contain vitamins and minerals, including vitamin D and calcium. Try mixing the three together for a great taste and increased nutritional benefits. This mixture tastes great on cereals, too.
- Begin replacing white breads with more nutritious options. Try the new 100 calorie sandwich rounds. They are made of whole grains and are filling and flavorful. Or try the bread that combines rye and pumpernickel in a swirl design—it looks fun and tastes great.
- Try soy products.
- Replace chicken stock with vegetable stock for soups and recipes.
- Try Meatless Mondays. This is a national public-health initiative that some restaurants are beginning to participate in.
- Replace a portion of the meats in your recipes with beans.
- Serve meat sauces rather than large meatballs or large pieces of beef.
- Visit your local farmers' market. Produce growers are eager to share their recipes for their products.

Eating more plant-based foods may be your most important baby step ever. You can do this. Pinch your excess fat once again, hopefully for the last time, and become a vegevore.

Vegevore Recipes

The following recipes are family favorites. They were chosen because they taste great and most important, you feel good about yourself right after eating them. They focus on fiber, grains, fruits, vegetables, and nuts. They also include small amounts of animal products if you choose.

Spinach Salad with Chicken

1 package baby spinach or spinach with mixed greens
4–6 ounces goat cheese, crumbled
1 cup dried cranberries
½ to 1 cup store-bought honey roasted/candied pecans
4 pieces cooked bacon strips
2 skinless, cooked chicken breasts cut into strips*

Raspberry vinaigrette dressing:
½ cup balsamic vinegar
¼ to ½ cup fresh or frozen raspberries
2 teaspoons sugar
Blend together above ingredients.

1. Combine spinach, cheese, cranberries, pecans and bacon. Top with chicken strips. Add raspberry vinaigrette dressing. This makes 3–4 servings.

*Store-bought roasted chicken is a time saver.

Whole Wheat Pizza

whole wheat pizza dough (store
  bought)
olive oil
pizza sauce, about 1 cup
mozzarella cheese, shredded

your choice of pizza toppings:
onions, peppers, mushrooms,
sausage, pepperoni, olives,
tomatoes, feta cheese,
pineapple, ham, etc. Be
creative!*

1. Follow instructions on whole wheat pizza dough.
2. Drizzle olive oil on large baking sheet pan. Spread dough to fit.
3. Drizzle olive oil on dough. Add pizza sauce, then cheese.
4. Add toppings.
5. Bake per package instructions.

*Adding raw onions, peppers, and mushrooms to the dough may result in soggy vegetables. Try sautéing them first. This will caramelize them which will also enhance their flavors. Also, note that thinly sliced pepperoni is only 10 calories per piece.

Harvest Soup with Lentils

2 tablespoons olive oil
1 clove garlic or 1 teaspoon
  garlic powder
1 onion, chopped
4 carrots, chopped
4 celery stalks, chopped
15 ounces tomato puree

2 cups chicken stock*
4 cups vegetable stock*
12 ounces red lentils
2 cups water
4–6 ounces pre-cooked smoked
  sausage cut into small pieces
  (optional)

1. In a large soup pot sauté onions, carrots, and celery in olive oil until tender. Add garlic and cook additional 1–2 minutes.
2. Add tomato puree, chicken stock and vegetable stock, lentils, and water. Bring to a boil. Cover and simmer 30 to 45 minutes until lentils are tender and soup has thickened, stirring occasionally. Add additional water if needed.
3. Add sausage.

This is a hearty, fulfilling soup that makes 8–10 servings. Serve with multi-grain bread.

*Low-salt chicken bouillon and vegetable bouillon can be substituted.

Honey-Pecan Chicken Fingers with Sweet & Spicy Sweet Potato Fries

Chicken Fingers:

1 egg
¼ cup honey
1 cup pecans (½ cup finely
   chopped, ½ cup ground)
½ cup bread crumbs
2–3 skinless chicken breasts cut
   into strips

1. Preheat oven to 375 degrees.
2. Beat egg and honey together. In separate dish, mix pecans and bread crumbs.
3. Dip chicken pieces in egg and honey mixture, then generously coat with pecan mixture.
4. Place on lightly greased baking pan and bake 30 minutes or until chicken is done.

Sweet & Spicy Sweet Potato Fries:

2 medium sweet potatoes,
   peeled and cut into ¼- to
   ½-inch strips
1 tablespoon canola oil
2 teaspoons brown sugar
2 teaspoons honey
½ teaspoon coriander
½ to 1 teaspoon chili powder

1. Preheat oven to 425 degrees.
2. Combine the sweet potatoes with the above ingredients. Roast the sweet potatoes on a baking sheet for about 18–22 minutes until crisp, turning once.

Serving suggestions: Serve with mixed greens.

Salmon with Molasses Sauce

$\frac{1}{4}$ cup molasses

$\frac{1}{4}$ cup coarse-grained mustard

2 tablespoons red wine vinegar

$\frac{3}{4}$ pound salmon fillets

1. Whisk together first 3 ingredients. Heat in saucepan until thickened, approx. 5–10 minutes.
2. Cook salmon in large skillet until almost done. Remove from skillet and remove fish skin.
3. Cut salmon into large pieces, add back to clean skillet. Add sauce and cook until salmon is done.

Serving suggestions: Serve over multi-grain rice with asparagus as a side dish. Serves 4.

Chili with Chicken and Chocolate

2 tablespoons olive oil
1 onion, chopped
3 cloves garlic, minced
1 tablespoon smoky ancho chile
    sauce*
1 tablespoon dried coriander
1 teaspoon paprika
1 teaspoon chili powder
¼ teaspoon cinnamon
2 cooked chicken breasts, skinless
    and cut into pieces

2 tablespoons tomato paste
1 cup chicken stock
15 ounces crushed tomatoes
1 can kidney beans, rinsed and
    drained
1 ounce bittersweet chocolate
    (not unsweetened)
1 cup cashews, optional

1. In a large heavy saucepan or Dutch oven cook onion in oil until softened. Add garlic and cook 1–2 minutes longer.

2. Add ancho chile sauce, coriander, paprika, chili powder, and cinnamon. Add chicken and stir to coat with mixture.

3. Stir in tomato paste, chicken stock, crushed tomatoes, and beans and simmer, covered, stirring occasionally to avoid sticking. Cook approx. 15 minutes until sauce is thickened. Add chocolate and cashews. Serve with multi-grain bread. Serves 4.

*I found this Mexican hot sauce in the international aisle of the supermarket sold under the Goya label as Salsita sauce.

Barley Soup with Swiss Chard and Sausage

1 tablespoon olive oil
2 carrots, chopped
1 onion, chopped
1 tablespoon tomato paste
2 cups low-sodium vegetable broth
2 cups low-sodium chicken broth

½ cup pearl barley
15 ounce can chickpeas, rinsed
1 bunch Swiss chard, chopped roughly
6 ounces cooked sausage (optional) cut into small pieces

1. In large soup pot heat olive oil and sauté carrots and onion until softened.
2. Add the tomato paste and cook, stirring, until it is slightly darkened, 1 to 2 minutes.
3. Add the vegetable broth and chicken broth, barley, and 2 cups water and bring to a boil. Reduce heat and simmer until barley is tender, 20 to 25 minutes. Add the Swiss chard, chickpeas, and sausage and simmer until the Swiss chard is tender, 5 minutes.

This hearty soup is a hit with kids. Show them the Swiss chard before cooking it. They will be excited to be cooking and eating such a colorful vegetable. Swiss chard is sold in giant bunches, sometimes including yellow, orange, and pink stems and leaves.

Turkey and Sweet Potatoes with Fruit Sauce

4 medium sweet potatoes
½ to 1 pound cooked turkey
    breast cut into pieces
2 tablespoons butter
½ cup currant jelly*
¼ cup orange juice

1 tablespoon lemon juice
1 lemon rind, grated
1 teaspoon dry mustard
1 teaspoon paprika
½ teaspoon ground ginger

1. Preheat the oven to 350 degrees.
2. Microwave sweet potatoes until tender.
3. Melt butter in saucepan. Stir in jelly, juices, and lemon rind. Add the spices, stirring to blend.
4. Arrange the turkey and sweet potatoes in a casserole dish and cover with ¾ cup of sauce.
5. Bake, uncovered, for approximately 30 minutes, basting occasionally with the remaining sauce.

*This recipe was originally tested using red currant jelly. I have also used 100% black currant fruit and 100% fruit mixtures; both tasted great.

Pasta Salad with Ham

½ cup mayonnaise
½ cup reduced-calorie sour cream
¼ cup mango chutney
12 ounces veggie pasta, cooked*
8 ounces baked ham, diced

1 cup diced carrots
1 cup diced celery
2 hard-cooked eggs, chopped
2 scallions, thinly sliced (both white and green parts)

Mix together mayonnaise, sour cream, and chutney. Combine with remaining ingredients in a large bowl.

*Pastas made with vegetables can be found in several shapes and sizes at most grocery stores.

Sweet and Sour "Mini" Meatballs

¼ cup brown sugar
1 tablespoon cornstarch
1 fresh pineapple cut into small
  chunks (about 1½ cups)
⅓ cup white vinegar
1 tablespoon soy sauce

1 red pepper, cut into large
  pieces
1 onion, cut into large pieces
1 cup snow peas or sugar snap
  peas (cooked)
½ cup cashews (optional)

1. Make ¾-inch round meatballs using ½ pound lean ground beef, or a mixture of ground beef and ground pork. Add garlic and onion for seasoning. (Use your family favorite recipe, just as long as you make "mini" sizes.)
2. Cook meatballs in skillet. Remove and drain excess fat. Mix brown sugar and cornstarch in skillet. Stir in pineapple, vinegar, and soy sauce. Heat to boiling, stirring constantly. Reduce heat. Add red pepper and onion and cook 5 minutes until slightly tender. Add back meatballs. Add snow peas and cashews just before serving. Serve 3–4 meatballs with brown rice per person.

25

Fall in Love with Nature's Bounty

Fruits and vegetables are nutritious and important to eat. **True**

Fruits and vegetables are viewed as accompaniments to your main food dish and are usually boring. **True**

Fruits and vegetables are cheap. **False**

If fruits and vegetables are so important, why are they considered ho-hum? There are hundreds of types of fruit and vegetables in the world. How can we be so bored?

Because fruits and vegetables are the #2 and #3 spots on our dinner plates, we tend to give them less attention. Being creative with the entire plate seven days a week can be a little daunting for most of us. Then there is the fact that these essential foods, which are nature's bounty, are costing us a fortune. A single piece of fruit can cost almost a dollar, the same with a single red pepper. It's in our best interests to change our perception of these accompaniments, however. We need to respect them and be grateful that we can afford and enjoy them.

I began thinking about how fine restaurants prepare and serve these accompaniments; they have to be original because their patrons expect the best. Chefs deliver by first enticing us with the presentation, then by taste. They use separate serving dishes, sauces, and garnishments to accomplish this. We can do this, too.

We all enjoy salads and fruit plates. The secret is to make them look like they were prepared by someone else, without all the fuss and cost. I started serving our fruit in small decorative bowls, and all of a sudden everyone noticed. I'd serve individual servings of salad on decorative glass plates and noticed a big change. I made a decorative fruit and vegetable platter with a dipping sauce, and the fingers and forks were flying! All I had to do was be a little creative and mix it up. I do not spend any real time or energy on this. My goal is only to add interest, not to become a celebrity chef. The bonus is that small decorative bowls and plates are plentiful and cheap at yard sales.

A single piece of fruit, such as a kiwi or an orange, looks beautiful plainly sliced and arranged on your dinner plate. It's simple and effective. We can all do this one.

Try adding yogurt and honey to your fruit dish. Start with ¼ cup of vanilla yogurt and add 1 tablespoon of honey. Add any combination of fruits and nuts that you enjoy, such as bananas, dark cherries, blueberries, walnuts, or pecans. This is a real crowd-pleaser, especially with the kids. It also helps to use up leftover fruit and nuts.

Let's all go back to nature and reassess our values. Look at fruits and vegetables as the incredible sources of vitamins and minerals that they are. They are as important as the main dish, and when presented in simple yet special ways, they are as enticing. They may be expensive, but they are essential. Fall in love with nature's bounty and enjoy. It is as simple as that.

Nature's Bounty: Fruit and Vegetable Recipes*

Red Grapefruit and Avocado Salad

¼–½ cup balsamic vinegar
1 teaspoon vegetable oil
1 tablespoon sugar

3 red grapefruits cut into sections
2 avocados cut into ¼-inch slices

In a large bowl, whisk together balsamic vinegar, oil, and sugar. Add grapefruit and avocados, tossing gently. Kids love this recipe.

Homemade Applesauce

8 assorted apples (e.g., Red Delicious, Empire, Braeburn, Granny Smith)*

1 cinnamon stick (optional)
½ cup apple cider or water

Peel, core, and cut the apples into large chunks. Cook in large, heavy saucepan, adding apple cider or water and cinnamon stick. Cook over med/high heat, covered, until apples are tender. Coarsely mash apples. Serve warm or chilled. Some people prefer to add ground cinnamon to individual servings after apples are cooked.

*Include both sweet and tart for great flavor

*These are all kid friendly!

Oven-Roasted Fruit

4 peaches, pitted and cut into quarters
4 plums, pitted and quartered
2 tablespoons sugar

1 cup fresh or frozen raspberries
2 tablespoons orange juice

1. Preheat the oven to 350 degrees.
2. Place the peaches and plums tightly in a single layer baking dish. Sprinkle with sugar and bake for 20 to 25 minutes until tender.
3. Cook the raspberries in a small pan. Strain out seeds. Add raspberry juice and orange juice to plums and peaches. Serve warm.

Makes 6 to 8 servings.

Mixed Vegetables

2 cups fresh or frozen corn (thawed)
1 cup edamame* found in fresh or frozen section

1 red pepper, diced
¼–½ cup balsamic vinegar
1 tablespoon sugar
1 teaspoon vegetable oil

Whisk together balsamic vinegar, sugar, and oil. Add to vegetables.

*Soybeans

Sweet Potatoes with Apples and Pears

4 Fuji apples*
3 Bartlett pears*
2–3 medium sweet potatoes

3 tablespoons butter or
    margarine
¼ cup brown sugar (or less)

1. Microwave sweet potatoes until tender.
2. Peel and core the apples and pears. Cut apples into large chunks and pears into ¼-inch wedges. Cook apples and pears in large skillet with butter until tender. Add cooked sweet potatoes and brown sugar. Serve warm.

*Experiment using your favorites.

Apple and Cranberry Cole Slaw

2 tablespoons maple syrup
1 tablespoon cider vinegar
⅓ cup mayonnaise
⅓ cup sour cream
3 cups shredded cabbage

1 cup dried cranberries
1 Granny Smith apple (with skin)
    cut into thin slices
1 Red Delicious apple (with skin)
    cut into thin slices

Stir together maple syrup, cider vinegar, mayonnaise and sour cream in large bowl. Mix in cabbage, cranberries and apples.

Roasted Bananas with Sweet Potatoes

This recipe tastes like a dessert!

2 bananas, unpeeled
3 medium sweet potatoes
¼ cup honey
½ cup almond flour

¼ stick butter, melted
¼ cup dark brown sugar
1 cup pecans, chopped

Preheat oven to 375 degrees.

1. Roast bananas in baking dish for 10 to 15 minutes until softened. (Skin will turn black.)
2. Microwave sweet potatoes for 10 to 15 minutes until softened.
3. Peel bananas and add to sweet potatoes with honey. Mix well.
4. In a separate bowl, mix flour, butter, brown sugar, and pecans.
5. Add topping and bake for about 20 minutes until golden.

Cold Berry Soup

2 cups fresh or frozen mixed
  berries (suggestions:
  strawberries, raspberries,
  blackberries, blueberries)*
2 tablespoons sugar

2 cups sparkling white grape
  juice, chilled
2 tablespoons sour cream
  (optional)

In a blender, puree berries with sugar. Strain out seeds if using raspberries. When ready to serve, add grape juice and sour cream. Serve immediately.

*Be creative with this recipe using a variety of berries and fruit. Also try non-alcoholic sparkling wine. This is a fun and delicious way to serve fruit. Serves 4.

26

Those Damn Calories.
It's Their Fault I'm Fat!

Calories, calories, calories.

Not only do your daily meals have to include 100 percent of the necessary vitamins and minerals, but they also must not go over your total allotted calories.

Yes, you have to go through your entire life counting calories. You can't go through life stuffing your face with whatever foods you like and continue to be clueless as to their calorie count. It's of utmost importance that you become knowledgeable about calories and become familiar with ingredient labels. It is critical for you to truthfully know if your lunch is actually several meals in one. You will also understand that desserts will most likely exceed your daily calories allowed (that is why they are desserts and not part of your meal). If you are informed, you will make better food choices, which will lead to being in control. Knowing the amount of calories in salad dressings and mayonnaise may make you think twice about how much you use.

We must pay attention to the appropriate sizes and amounts to meet, not exceed, our daily caloric intake. Let's learn the basics of calorie counting for once and for all.

Each pound of body fat equals 3,500 calories. It doesn't matter whether you eat 3,500 calories of healthy foods or 3,500 calories of unhealthy foods; it's still the same amount of calories. It can't be any simpler. If you want to lose a pound, you have to delete 3,500 calories from your body. This is one diet fact that no one disputes.

This is why there are so many crash diets. People choose to eat one food item because either it is low in calories or they love it and eat only enough calories to just survive. You know the diets, and we all know how these diet scenarios turn out.

Before you actually count calories, you will need a guide to esti-mate the number of calories that you need. There are several sources, including the USDA website, that will help you determine this. The calculation includes your age and amount of daily exercise. After inputting this, you can then determine how many calories you can safely eliminate each day to obtain your goal. Be sure to check with your doctor or nutritionist before you begin your plan.

I'll never forget one summer vacation several years ago. We were at an ice cream stand at the beach, deciding which flavors we each wanted. While we were deciding, a woman with a trim figure approached the counter asking about the number of calories in the ice cream. She then proceeded to ask how many calories were in the frozen yogurt. She pondered over the answers given her, thanked the staff, and then decided not to buy either. As she walked away, I heard snickering from several people, including myself. You've got to be kidding: counting calories during the summer while at the beach? I knew the lesson here, but I did not connect the dots until much later.

Common Foods	Calories
1 tablespoon mayonnaise	100
1 tablespoon mustard	16
1 tablespoon ketchup	16
1 tablespoon sour cream	26
1 tablespoon salted butter	100
1 tablespoon vegetable oil	120
1 tablespoon whipped cream	8
1 tablespoon heavy cream	51
1 teaspoon sugar	16
Salad dressings: 2 tablespoons	
French	140
Blue Cheese	130
Italian	140
12 ounces soda, cola	140
8 ounces whole milk	150
8 ounces skim milk	86
1 slice white bread	100
1 egg	80
1 slice (1 ounce) American cheese	106

Counting calories is actually easier than you think. Once you familiarize yourself with calorie charts, you will see how you can become pretty good at estimating the calories of a particular food. One way to do this is to keep a small calories booklet in your kitchen.

As you review your calorie-counting source, notice the patterns: most vegetables and fruits have low amounts of calories in the recommended portion sizes. Because of this, I consider most vegetables and fruits as freebies. I eat as much salad greens, peppers, onions, apples, peaches, and grapes as I want. Note that 3 to 4 ounces is the recommended portion size for your meats, chicken, and fish. It should now become apparent to you that most restaurant portions are quite large.

Look for the specific foods in every category that have the highest amount of calories per portion size. High-caloric amounts do not mean you should skip these foods. You just need to evaluate these foods as to their importance to your diet and adjust the amounts of each accordingly.

Familiarizing yourself with counting calories is very important. Every weight-loss program must eventually end, and you will have to fend for yourself. If you know your calories, eating food at restaurants will no longer be a calorie guessing game. You will already know the basics. Some restaurants, including fast-food restaurants, even post these numbers for all to see. No longer should you order that sandwich because of its abundant size. You will know whether it is a single meal or two sandwiches in one. You'll think twice about nonstop, uncontrolled eating.

Do not look at calorie counting as a spoiler to your eating pleasure. It is a lifelong guide to your wellbeing, along with your kids' and pets'. Look at this knowledge as power that will lead to more informed and better choices.

Knowing the basics of food and their calorie counts is a key to good eating habits. I am pleased that nutrition classes still exist and are an important part of my children's school curriculum. Good work, teachers!

27

Let's Talk About Poop

inally—a fun topic to talk about!

I've always believed that you shouldn't even consider being a parent until you experience caring for a baby for at least a week. You will learn that pooping is an important function that parents have to pay close attention to. Not because diapers are gross and have to be changed often, but because this bodily function is an important part of one's health. The color, size, and texture of each poop reflects a person's nutrition intake. You literally have to analyze your child's poop throughout his or her development, not just at the baby stage. Who knew you would have to be a potty monitor?

The same applies to pets. Don't even consider getting a large dog unless you are capable of being a responsible dog owner by picking up and disposing of your dog's daily poop. And I don't meant tying the poop bag around your dog's leash so he has to carry his own excrement. Can you believe some owners actually do this? Big dogs need to exercise just as humans do to keep their systems regular. This means a decent walk every day. And a well-fed, exercised large dog could mean several large poops a day.

Why on earth do you have to monitor a dog's poop? We feed our family dog, Ginger Rose, twice a day and thus twice a day she poops. If she does not have two sessions in one day, she will have to go out sometime during the night or she will have an accident in the house. If her stools are not lovely formed shapes, then she, too, might be suffering from poor nutrition or physical ailments. Yes, pooping is a big deal.

OK, back to humans and their poop. Back in high school, I remember a science teacher giving a lecture on this. He stated that the act of pooping is actually a pleasurable physical experience when your system is in good working order. Oh, my. Too much information. Although I'll never forget that lecture because of its over-sharing, it does help remind me of the importance of a balanced diet.

Do your body an immense favor by adding more fiber to your meals. You probably glossed over that last sentence because you've heard it a million times. I even bored myself by writing it.

Let's try again. The National Institutes of Health (NIH) recommends the following fiber sources: oat bran, barley, nuts, seeds, beans, lentils, peas, wheat bran, whole grains, and some fruits and vegetables. Some serving-size suggestions and basic nutrition facts appear on the next page.

How many grams of fiber do adults need for a pleasurable pooping experience? The NIH recommends 20 grams to 35 grams per day for adults. The beauty of fiber is that it is in the everyday foods we eat and enjoy. Look at the suggestions on the next page; they are not weird or unusual foods and they are very low in calories.

It is recommended that you add fiber gradually to your diet to

Food	Serving Size	Total Fiber (grams)	Calories
Grains			
oatmeal	1 cup	4.0	145
pearled barley, cooked	1 cup	6.0	200
brown rice	1 cup	3.5	216
multigrain bread	1 slice	1.9	70
whole wheat spaghetti	1 cup	6.2	170
Beans, Nuts, Seeds			
lentils, cooked	1 cup	15.6	215
black beans, cooked	1 cup	15.0	200
split peas, cooked	1 cup	16.3	230
almonds	1 oz. (24 nuts)	3.5	165
pecans	1 oz. (19 halves)	2.7	190
sunflower seed kernels	¼ cup	3.9	160
Fruits & Vegetables			
raspberries	1 cup	8.0	60
pear with skin	1 medium	5.1	100
strawberries	1 cup	3.3	60
banana	1 medium	3.1	105
sweet potato, cooked	1 cup	5.9	180
pumpkin, canned, cooked	1 cup	7.0	40
broccoli, cooked	1 cup	5.1	19

avoid abdominal discomfort and that you drink plenty of fluids to aid the passage of fiber through the digestive system.

Note, too, that by changing your morning eating ritual (chapter 19), you will add valuable fiber to your eating plan.

28

I Am Going to Make You Cry

*T*his one is going to hurt: you can't have desserts every day. Ouch! Desserts are a touchy subject. The U.S. is a "dessertaholic" society. Children are given desserts as a bribe to finish their dinners. Adults feel entitled to them. Why must we always have something sweet after a meal? The meal itself should be enough. Why is one accused of dieting if one refuses dessert? Worse yet, you are insulting your host if you dare to say you are too full for dessert. And let's not forget that offer of a second piece so nothing goes to waste. I think that line was first delivered by the devil himself. In fact, we sometimes eat our meals like ravenous wild boars just to get to that dessert. Why on earth do we feel entitled to eat high-calorie, fattening foods every day?

Dessert has become the high point of the meal. People can't recall what you served them for dinner, but they'll always remember dessert. Prospective brides and grooms take note: Forget about shelling out big bucks for extravagant dinners at your wedding. Go straight for the cake!

This brings to mind an episode of *Roseanne* centered on the family's attempt to diet. The husband refused to give up his food, including desserts and alcohol, because, by golly, they don't have much else in life. I can picture the majority of TV viewers yelling "Hallelujah!" at that moment.

Going out to dinner is always a battle. Restaurants have dessert and specialty-drink marketing down to a science. They suggest them at the beginning of the order-taking, when you are most vulnerable. You have seen the appealing fliers at your table, and if your children are present, the servers know that parents will cave when it comes to making their kids happy with dessert. Some restaurants really fire the big guns at you at the end of the meal by presenting the famous dessert tray for all to see. You may as well surrender at this point. You are the ultimate party pooper at your dinner table if you refuse dessert now.

I know that my kids secretly declare me the worst mom on the planet when we eat at restaurants. I do not allow any of us to over-indulge on desserts at this time. I want us to enjoy our meals, not the notion that an ooey, gooey dessert is waiting at the end. No matter how I try to present my case, I know that I will never be voted Mom of the Year. I just remain firm on this issue, determined to prevail. We are always full from our meals and dessert would be food overload. Money also plays a factor. Restaurant meals are a luxury. When the kids demand desserts too, it becomes a budget buster for me. Whether my teenagers agree with me or not, at least for now they are restraining themselves from stabbing me with their forks.

Of course, we do enjoy desserts. I just try to keep them separate from our main meals. We love ice cream parlors and occasional trips to dessert cafés.

We also have a weekly dessert compromise: I let our girls choose two days a week when they can have their "snack nights." They chose Tuesday and Friday. They love ice cream, so they pick their favorite and I just nonchalantly monitor portion sizes. This works for us because it makes two days a week special. To offset the other days we do keep a candy jar filled with bite-sized chocolates, allowing everyone to select one or two pieces. These miniature chocolates are satisfying and contain a fraction of the calories that regular-sized candy bars contain. This candy jar is a real necessity because my younger daughter is such a chocoholic that I worry for my safety. Besides, eating a small amount of chocolate each day does make the world seem a better place.

Desserts are special. Don't make them an ordinary part of your meal. Desserts during vacations and celebrations are well-deserved indulgences. Break loose and have ice cream for lunch as a special treat? You betcha!

29

Nonstop Eating Is the Way to Go!

*T*here is a new philosophy regarding eating habits that is gaining national attention. The focus is on eating smaller meals, more often.

It is bizarre that we eat three large meals a day, with five to six hours in between lunch and dinner. Think about this for a few minutes. We are all ravenous by 3 P.M., and we need food. We accept that school kids do, but most adults look for food about this time also. Just picture all the workers who suddenly appear at the office vending machine in the late afternoon. That is why it is there in the first place. We are so hungry that we grab anything in sight to satisfy our hunger pangs. Imagine all the unnecessary calories due to this starvation-type eating. Imagine what this odd-structured eating does to our blood sugar levels.

Now that I'm going through menopause, my hormones are going berserk. It is not the hot flashes I am concerned with. Those I can handle. It is the sudden wave of feeling nauseous without warning that annoys me. I never vomit, I just feel as if I need to. My doctor confirmed that my body was experiencing hormonal changes, and to alleviate my symptoms, she recommended this new way of eating. Eat more often, in smaller portions, and include proteins. It really works for me.

Every couple of hours I'll eat something that includes cheese, an egg, yogurt, nuts, or a soy drink. I eat real foods, not low-calorie or dietetic foods. Because I am eating a smaller meal doesn't mean I want to compromise taste or quality. I monitor my portion sizes, ever so aware of the calorie content. Sometimes I'll divide my lunch in two and have two lunches. I also keep a small bag of mixed fruit and nuts in my purse at all times, especially for travel.

This change has brought me tremendous relief because I didn't choose hormone replacement therapy. I want to keep all my body parts functioning at optimum levels throughout the day, and eating smaller portions of great-tasting foods that meet my personal needs works for me.

It works for teens, too. My daughters participated in high school sports this year. With the players practicing two hours a day, the coaches emphasized how important it was for them to keep up their energy level by eating more nutritious foods. She also recommended that they eat throughout the day, not just at lunch time or at the end of school before practice begins. I thought this was excellent, innovative advice.

I have often asked my teenagers if teachers allowed eating and drinking in class to compensate for those who have earlier or later lunches. Ask your kids about their school lunchtimes; if they start at 8 A.M. and the first lunch is at 10:30, then it's an awfully long time before dinner. Eating during the last lunchtime will lead to hunger pangs during the long morning session, as well as during the afternoon until dinnertime.

Parents and schools are doing a great job of getting rid of junk foods in vending machines and lunches, but what about maintaining students' energy levels throughout the day? My daughters tell me that water is always allowed and that kids munch on foods as they are travelling between classes. There shouldn't be a free-for-all when it comes to food and drink, but it does make sense to allow some type of eating regimen throughout the day that doesn't disrupt the class.

In case you didn't notice, I have not used the word *snack*. Snacks equate to foods that temporarily fulfill you and may not be very nutritious. Snacks are meant to bully you away from the real meal that you want but can't have because the clock says so. Most of the weight-loss plans that sell packaged meals include snacks to take the edge off of the hunger. These snacks are pretend versions of the food we really want. Some have dietetic sugars, skimpy sizes, and odd chocolate flavorings. They are not exactly yummy. I am embarrassed for the celebrities who claim they actually like these snacks. Fine, let's watch them eat them for the rest of their lives.

Common sense tells us that not giving our bodies fuel for five to six hours while our engines are still running is not sensible behavior. Nonstop eating in smaller portions is the way to go. Let's give more attention to this new food philosophy.

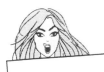

30

Stop Bastardizing Chocolate!

Stop bastardizing chocolate, and just eat the real stuff already. No one should make or eat anything but the pure, indulgent, intoxicating stuff. Get rid of anything that pretends to look or feel like chocolate. If it is not the good stuff, don't eat it. Why would you waste precious calories on fake or modified chocolate? Chocolate is too important in our lives, so don't mess with it.

Don't waste your time looking at a product that surrounds itself in chocolate as a marketing gimmick. Know the difference between adding chocolate to enhance a product and adding it to disguise a

> "Chocolate is nature's way of making up for Mondays."
> —Anonymous
>
> "All I really need is love, but a little chocolate now and then doesn't hurt!"
> —Lucy Van Pelt in *Peanuts* by Charles M. Schultz

"I have this theory that chocolate slows down the aging process. . . . It may not be true, but do I dare take the chance?"

—Author Unknown

"Exercise is a dirty word. . . . Every time I hear it, I wash my mouth out with chocolate."

—Author Unknown

"Giving chocolate to others is an intimate form of communication, a sharing of deep, dark secrets."

—Milton Zelma

product. Selling chocolate-flavored foods may be a brilliant marketing plan, but I do not want my kids to be fooled. I want my kids to eat foods because they know that they are made of nutritious stuff and are even fortified with vitamins and minerals, not because they are disguised to look or taste like dessert. This is not a helpful parenting trick for me.

Adding chocolate to a product makes the item a dessert, so you might as well have a piece of chocolate cake instead. I actually threw a hissy fit in the grocery store over this. I was so frustrated that my young kids were always begging me to get any products on the shelves that contained chocolate, especially some of the cereals, that one day I just screamed, "Go ahead and just eat chocolate for breakfast, lunch, and dinner every day!" A woman in the same aisle laughed out loud, but then she told me that I was absolutely correct.

And forget about substitute chocolate desserts to try to satisfy your sweet tooth. Yuck. Life is definitely too short for that nonsense. Trying to cover the world in chocolate may sound like nirvana, but it only dilutes the pleasure of chocolate.

Keep chocolate as the aphrodisiac that it is meant to be. You can eat real decadent chocolate and still lose weight. Calculate the

> "I could give up chocolate but I'm not a quitter."
> —Author Unknown

> "Make a list of important things to do today. At the top of your list, put 'eat chocolate.' Now you'll get at least one thing done today."
> —Gina Hayes

> "Chemically speaking, chocolate really is the world's perfect food."
> —Michael Levine

> "I don't understand why so many so called chocolate lovers complain about the calories in chocolate, when all true chocoholics know that it is a vegetable. It comes from the cocoa bean, beans are veggies, 'nuff said."
> —Author Unknown

number of calories that your favorite pieces of chocolate contain, and incorporate them into your plan. You may have to make choices, so be sensible. A great idea is to keep bite-sized candy available to eat throughout the day. M&M's are a wonderful choice; a few of these throughout the day satisfies my chocolate cravings. I also cut large chocolate bars into pieces and then strategically eat them at different times of the day. I can eat nutritious meals and have chocolate every day. How great is that?

"Man cannot live on chocolate alone; but woman sure can."

—Author Unknown

Go to the website: www.sassy-gal.com to see a daily chocolate quote!

31

"Bad to the Bone" Foods

Oh, those delicious, sinfully bad-to-the-bone foods that we must have—the foods that we dream about and the foods we can't live without. Those foods that cause cravings, temptations, and food highs that are the ultimate failure of all diets. These are the foods that give us immediate pleasure and condition our brain to crave them over and over. We have been lectured to death on how we must stop eating foods that are not good for us.

These are the foods that the devil uses to sabotage us and therefore must be eliminated from our lives completely. Here is where I hold my fingers to form the sign of the cross and stand up to the devil. He will not win this one.

I can't be told to eliminate chocolate, potato chips, pizza, and soft drinks from my life. I refuse to give them up, and I don't have to. People start and stop these restrictive diets over and over because the diets are unrealistic. Food deprivation equals punishment, which leads to failure. Cravings are your body screaming at you that it needs or wants something. You think you can satisfy your chocolate craving with a piece of sugar-free chocolate? Maybe temporarily. But your body knows the difference, and it is only a matter of time before you cave and gorge yourself with the chocolate you wanted in the first place. No secret there. This technique is sure to lead to another diet failure.

Finding a substitute for the food you really want to help you take the edge off is preposterous. Unless you are tied up with duct tape over your mouth, your body (influenced by the devil, of course) will eventually lead you to that food, and then make you overeat to punish you for trying to fool it. So be truthful about what you truly crave, and then see how you can incorporate it into your food plan.

According to the USDA, there is room in your daily calorie intake for "discretionary calories." These include foods that are mostly fats or sweeteners, including candy and alcohol.

This does not give you permission to indulge every whim, however. You will have to analyze (or get help analyzing) the total number of calories you can allot to these types of foods. These foods are also not a replacement for the necessary food groups you need but a supplement for your enjoyment. Make sure your food craving choices are legitimate and not an excuse to add unnecessary calories, including excess alcohol or outrageous combinations of fatty, salty, or sugary foods.

Only you can determine what gives you your food high, so be honest here. No matter what it is, declare it, analyze it, and try to incorporate it into your life.

Use the following chart to declare to yourself for once and all when you snack to excess, sneak foods, eat as a distraction, and pretend not to eat while you are eating (eat while doing a second activity,

Food Cravings

	Food	Calories	Nutritional Value
Morning			
Afternoon			
Evening			
Late Night			

like watching TV). Then list the foods that you absolutely must have in your life, including their calorie amounts and nutritional value. You may need to make a separate chart for the weekend if your eating habits are significantly different.

In chapter 26 we learned how to calculate the average daily required calories to maintain our individual weight. An important factor in determining these calories is the level of your daily physical activity. Summarize these findings with your food cravings and determine how many of your food cravings can be classified as discretionary calories. For those who are not physically active, the discretionary calorie allowances are small, around 100 to 300 calories. A person who walks for 40 minutes at a brisk pace (4 mph) will burn between 149 and 220 calories, possibly allowing for more discretionary calories. People who participate in sports, dance, and certain types of exercise can burn off even more calories, which will lead to a greater number of discretionary calories.

Also determine the nutritional value of each item to further analyze how much you can incorporate into your plan. In other words, are your food cravings beneficial or junk foods? Chapter 2 3 will help you.

Important: Separate your food cravings from your bad food behaviors. For example, I love to dip my pizza crusts into creamy blue cheese dressing. This definitely is a bad food behavior for me. The slice of pizza is sufficient to meet my food craving. Adding the blue cheese dressing is being piggy because it just adds additional calories from fat, which I don't need.

32

Sweet-Salty-Sweet-Salty: The Sugar-Salt Roundabout

Sometimes I feel as if I'm psychotic. One moment I want something sweet, the very next moment, I want something salty. I have endured this phenomenon as long as I can remember.

While working at a former job, I had a jar of M&M's on my desk and a bag of potato chips in my desk. I knew at a young age that when I craved one, I would certainly crave the other within a short time. I figured there must be a scientific explanation for this phenomenon, of which hormones must be a factor, but I didn't care to know the specifics. Each afternoon I would indulge in a few of each to satisfy my cravings, and that was that.

I did eventually research this topic to get the facts once and for all. Alas, there is no simple answer. I found references to mood states, biological factors, gender differences, psychological factors, spiritual connectedness, food deprivation, dehydration, and even social pressure. It's certainly a complex matter.

In keeping with my "just move forward" approach, I'll avoid all scientific hypotheses here. There is a lot of research on food cravings, and I don't wish to overanalyze anything relating to dieting that is not life-threatening to me. Besides, here is not where I overindulge. I truly have just a few pieces of chocolate and a couple of chips.

On the other hand, if you find yourself out of control regarding this sugar-salt roundabout, then investigate it further. There are explanations galore, and I don't care what they are. I know the phenomenon exists, and acknowledging this sugar-salt craving helps me from racing toward that full bag of chips right after I've had a piece of chocolate. Since I enjoy both, I make sure there is room for both in my game plan.

33

Your Weight and the Big Body Theory

Weigh Yourself

Pay attention to your weight. Gaining a couple of pounds may be OK, but five pounds is not.

Only you know exactly how your body looks in your underwear and how you feel about it. Don't believe others when they say you are already thin when you've chosen the right clothes to hide that excess fat. Be truthful with yourself. Know that even your best friend will lie to you. You know how fat your butt really is. You have to keep an eye on your exact weight to keep it under control.

Mirrors Sometimes Lie

Mirrors don't always reflect back your true body shape. We have all discovered how different mirrors can be while clothes shopping. Maybe you just ignore that image in front of you, your mind playing an ingenious game to try to protect you. Maybe the devil's reflection is staring back at you from the mirror, whispering hauntingly, "You look great! Have a piece of cake!"

How many times have you heard someone say that the person in the mirror couldn't possibly be them? They just don't want to believe that those flabby arms or chubby face is theirs. Take a picture of yourself in your bathing suit or underwear. Then be prepared to see the truth and believe what you see.

Understand the Big Body Theory

Take out your high school yearbook, and notice how you and your friends have physically changed over the years. I am not talking about weight gain but about body shape. Look at how small your body frame seems compared to now. I call this the Big Body Theory. Our body frames have widened, including our heads. We all know that certain parts of our bodies keep growing, such as our ears and noses. Really look at how you have filled out, especially your face. Our bodies seem to have transformed into adult bodies even if we have not gained extra fat. Our basic skeletal frames seem bigger. Look at old family photos, too, and you'll see what I mean.

Most experts agree that it is normal to gain 10 pounds to 15 pounds as you grow past your youth, and you most likely can't lose it.

The last damn 10 pounds means whatever your individual acceptable weight should be and that you can maintain. It is not those pounds that will turn back the clock to make you a teenager again.

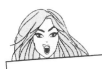

34

Let's Cook!

Television programs are a wonderful resource for new recipes and cooking instruction. Watch TV chefs and familiarize yourself with the chefs that really respect food—those who teach quality over quantity when preparing their recipes. Quality means pure, simple flavors, not foods drenched in grease, butter, or sauces. Notice especially how they orchestrate dishes. Do they prepare foods to enhance flavors, or do they hide the flavors with nonessential fats? Should their shows be called "Cooking with Butter"? Do they gently arrange meals on plates and proudly serve them, or do they glob piles onto the plate and scream, "Eat and get out!"?

Internet food sites also offer us an abundance of recipes to try. They often include such details as calories per serving size, salt and fat contents, and nutritional value, all of which will help us choose healthy meals.

I appreciate the attention given to our changing attitudes about how food should be prepared and how it should taste. The days of over-saucing, over-salting, and over-buttering are over. The simple, natural taste of foods that are locally produced is all the rage. Organically grown foods are becoming more popular and more readily available. Plus the abundance of new fruits and vegetables and whole wheat and whole grain products is incredible.

Here are some tidbits for adding flavor without the excess fat, salt, or sugar:

- **Vegetables:** Vegetables can be completely transformed with simple changes and without adding extra calories. Oven-roasting several vegetables together with a splash of olive oil and a sprinkle of seasonings is a simple method, yet it creates extremely flavorful results because of the caramelization.
- **Fruits:** Also consider oven-roasting several fruits together to enhance their natural flavors. Adding raspberries (which have been simmered with water and reduced) to the fruits after roasting will add even more flavor.
- **Oil-and-vinegar salad dressing:** Change the oil:vinegar ratio. Instead of using 3 tablespoons of oil and 1 tablespoon cider vinegar, reverse it. Using just 1 tablespoon of oil will dramatically change the flavor of your dressing. You can add a little sugar to cut the vinegar's acidity. Your salad will taste fresher and less oily. Not only are you decreasing the amount of oil in your dressing, but you are also increasing the flavor. You must try this one.
- **Sautéing:** Decrease the amount of butter and oil used when sautéing. You actually need very little of either to keep food from sticking to the pan and to caramelize the food. Why on earth

would you cover your food in a half inch of oil to cook it? Do not copy television chefs in this. They use extra oils for visualization only, and they over-use oils and butters in some recipes. I actually watched a TV celebrity chef's guest cringe when he saw how much butter the chef was adding to his mashed potatoes. The guest practically said, "Yuck."

- **Whole wheat pizza:** Store-bought whole wheat pizza dough is delicious and easy. Some whole wheat products aren't that flavorful, but whole wheat dough tastes great. It's also easy to prepare. You don't need to spin it in the air to create that perfect circle for your round pizza pan. Just stretch the dough to fit any large, shallow rectangular cooking sheet that has been lightly greased with olive oil. Add the toppings of your choice, and bake according to the package instructions. Create your own pizzas for family fun night.
- **Steamed fresh or frozen vegetables:** No one likes soggy vegetables. Don't boil vegetables in water when steaming is an option. Adults and kids really do enjoy vegetables when they are prepared correctly.
- **Brown sugar and butter:** Don't automatically add these to vegetables. This is an ingrained habit for some of us. Sugar pumpkin tastes great alone. The goal is to enhance the natural flavor of food, not taste sugar and butter. This is what is meant by clean, wholesome-tasting food.
- **Olive oil:** Use olive oil for more health benefits. Just remember that certain varieties of olive oil may taste bitter to some palates. Experiment with your recipes. You don't have to give up that

delicious garlic shrimp over linguine. Just adjust the olive oil and butter to more reasonable levels. Oils shouldn't have to be dripping down your chin for a dish to be a favorite.

- **Coconut oil:** Explore the new research on coconut oils for its benefits and for cooking. Try out recipes that feature coconut oil.
- **Sugar:** Sugar is not forbidden. Adding a small amount to fresh berries and other fruit brings out their natural juices, enhancing the flavor. One teaspoon of sugar is only 16 calories. Kids will appreciate this one; they like to drink the excess juices.
- **Salt:** Do not add salt to pasta water. This is not where we want to season our food. You want to taste the pasta and sauce, not salty pasta.

I am thrilled that we no longer base our cooking solely on one historic cookbook and our traditional family recipes. We can experiment, and we can teach new methods to our children so that they, too, can be creative while eating healthy. The entire world of cooking is literally at our fingertips. The resources available to us are endless, so take this free knowledge and prepare meals that your family will thrive on and enjoy. They are counting on you to do what is best for them and you.

35

Dinnertime Blues

*L*et's face it, your family does not run to the dinner table for that once-a-day face time and great conversation. They are in it for the food.

I noticed that what we were having for dinner was delivering immediate joy or disappointment to my family. I swear, some nights I even drove my husband and kids straight to depressionville. Dinner should not have to meet such high expectations. I am trying the best I can to work, clean, listen, chauffeur, encourage, help, hug, move us all forward, and keep the dog happy. Am I supposed to be a five-star chef as well? Dinner should not be a daily reward for a day's work, and if it is, it shouldn't be at Mom's (or Dad's) expense.

Add to this fact that you are trying to lose weight. Unless the whole gang is trying to lose weight, you have a challenge for yourself. To alleviate the dinnertime blues, try a few of the following suggestions. Making your family a part of the process takes the pressure off you and can even add some fun to dinnertime. We have a win-win.

- **Make one night a week salad bar night.** Everyone makes their own salad, adding chicken, steak, salmon, shrimp, or whatever protein you like. If choosing oil and vinegar for the salad dressing, remember to use the new ratio (1 Tbsp. oil to 3 Tbsp. cider vinegar). Varying the ingredients is key. Try avocados, beans, nuts, and cheese. Here is a great place to add those 15-plus types of beans and numerous vegetables that you don't have a clue what else to do with.
- **Once a month is finger food night.** This is fun food night. Whole wheat pizzas or chicken wings (baked, of course) work great here. It's an easy meal, and everyone can help.
- **Once a week is soup or sandwich night.** Homemade soups are such comfort foods, and when made with low-salt broths, the calorie content can be quite low. Try using vegetable stock. This is also the best place to add nutritious breads. The variety of whole wheat and multigrain breads and rolls supplied by your local stores are a real timesaver. Sandwiches are another crowd pleaser. Try panini (grilled sandwiches) or tea sandwiches (sandwiches cut into quarters). A cup of soup and a half sandwich combination is a good option for leftover soup. This idea is easier than you might think and is fun.
- **Once a week have vegetarian night.** This may be a bit more challenging, but the rewards are worth the effort. Soups, such as lentil, 15-bean (the beans come prepackaged), and vegetable, work well here. The idea is not so much to replace meats in your meals but to add more options, including vegetables.
- **Friday night is fish night.** Make your own fish and chips night by preparing a simple salmon dinner, crab cakes, grilled tuna,

or cod fish and adding oven-baked french fries as a side dish. I was thrilled when chipotle sauce was introduced; it is a fantastic accompaniment for crab cakes. You can buy it at any supermarket.

- **Eat more turkey.** For some reason, we treat turkey as a special-occasion food, limiting the number of times per year we serve it. This should not be the case. Turkey is inexpensive and tastes great. You can even purchase a precooked turkey breast to make preparation easy. Add different side dishes, maybe a different type of dressing. Add purchased orange-cranberry relish to create a complete new turkey dinner. And don't forget our favorite: turkey sandwiches. This is the time to experiment with your turkey dishes, not during the holidays. Keep your favorite turkey and side-dish recipes for your holiday traditions.

- **Make one night a week leftover night.** I am not talking about leftovers from the previous night's meal. I am talking about a Thursday or Friday when you have odds and ends left over from several days. Your family can eat what they want and when. Just guide the kids on this one, and everyone can have a relaxing dinner night.

Create a cheat sheet listing your most-loved recipes and tape it to the inside of a cabinet door. This is a real timesaver. I found that getting out my recipe books for ideas or aimlessly surfing the Internet took too long. Save this time for your weekly meal planning or for a special occasion.

Get your family involved, be creative, and have fun getting rid of the dinnertime blues.

36

The Four-Pig Restaurant Rating System

By the time Friday arrives, I am tired of planning and cooking meals. Weekends are for rejuvenating of our spirits, and we are on reprieve from our weekly big kitako removal. Let the fun begin! Be gone, weekly drudgery; restaurants, here we come!

Before we make that reservation, though, we must find the compromise needed to satisfy all our food senses without feeling angry at ourselves because we waddled out of the restaurant. Forget four-star ratings, try the four-pig rating system to determine how much we can eat at each restaurant.

First, think about what type of restaurant you are going to. Is it a culinary delight, with everything from appetizers to dessert being extraordinary? Is it a good restaurant where the main dishes are savored or dessert is a specialty? Is it a fun place to enjoy a burger, fries, and drink, or is it a diner type where comfort food is king? (Note: I am not talking about fast-food joints.)

Next, consider the décor and location of the restaurant. Is it white table cloth and candlelight? Beach front? Is dancing the attraction? Is it a club? Maybe it's just a comfortable place to hang out.

Now, think of why you are going to the restaurant and assign pigs to it. Note that this system is reversed, where the fewer pigs assigned, the better.

1 pig

You are invited to a top-rated, exceptional restaurant for a celebration. If you are a guest, sample everything that is offered. Never pass up something of this quality that is free. The experience of dining at a high-caliber establishment is a luxury that will intoxicate all your senses for quite some time. I believe a few extra calories here are meaningless. If you are paying for your dining experience, bring home a doggy bag so that you can extend the pleasure to another day (and spread out the calories).

2 pigs

When the location is the attraction, let the sights and sounds fill your soul. Eat moderately and enjoy the surroundings. Now is not the time to order five courses. You are overindulging for no reason. The location is your entertainment, not the food. Only the restaurants say that you have to order appetizers and dessert. The more food and drinks, the happier the customer, they preach. Don't buy into it; it just equals a bigger check. Ignore the server's badgering about all the extras. As long as you don't overstay your welcome and you spend an appropriate amount per person, you are OK. Enjoy the view and the company. Enjoy your food and drink—slowly. Go home feeling good about how grand the scenery was. The food should be secondary.

3 pigs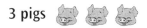

If the evening is all about drinks and dancing, the food should be minimal. Consume your main meal beforehand, and don't overindulge in the finger foods and "piggy martinis." Remember that those calories would be considered in the dessert or snack category and are possibly excessive. If everyone is dancing the Macarena or grinding on the dance floor and you're not because you can't drag yourself away from the snack bar, then you are at the wrong event. You may as well be home on the couch, watching TV and snorting like a pig when the food commercials come on.

4 pigs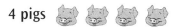

These restaurants are the most dangerous because comfort food rules here. Soft drinks are endless and you get fries, fries, and more fries with everything. Even the macaroni and cheese comes with fries. And let's not even talk about the entire deep-fried menu that comes with fries. We all love these restaurants, so what do we do?

This is a tough one because the restaurants cater to families and singles who want a casual night out without spending a fortune. You know the restaurants that I mean. They serve familiar foods, but add a twist to them. The food may be a slight upgrade from your average midweek meal, just enough more than what you would prepare at home so you won't be disappointed. The décor is fun, the atmosphere is comfortable, and the prices are midrange to hit that mass market. What a perfect marketing strategy for them, but not such a great deal for us.

Sure, we are fed big portions at a reasonable price, but next time take a good look at your check. This average restaurant has really just sucked every dollar it could out of you because you started with that special drink and appetizer and ended with dessert. And the calories! These were calories from average foods: were they worth it? All we wanted was a night off from cooking to enjoy a meal in a fun, casual setting. It was more expensive than we thought, both in money and wasted calories. And to think most of us frequent these places often. Maybe we should spend a little more on less-frequent, special meals. Ouch! I think Grandma just hit me over the head with her fry pan finally waking me with this lesson.

And those hometown diners and favorite family hangouts? They deserve 1 pig, if done infrequently. An occasional get-together with friends at that cozy diner is surely worth the calories. The memories you make with your family and friends are priceless. Just eat with your left hand if you are right-handed. I've heard that changing hands will confuse the brain into not knowing how to count calories.

37

Guiding Your Kids: Don't Be a Parenting Fool

As a parent, I am most proud of my attempt to guide my two girls toward commonsense eating. I never said, "Eat so and so because it is good for you." I always stated how good something tasted instead. I would casually mention why we ate so many types of fruits and vegetables, ad-libbing as I talked. I never wanted to sound like a doctor lecturing them, so I made explanations up as I went along. On one occasion, I told my young daughters that peas were good for your fingertips. Silly, I know, but as I wiggled my fingertips at them, they giggled and happily munched on their peas, wiggling their own fingertips.

Don't be the parent who believes that kids hate vegetables. Of course they like vegetables! It's common knowledge that it takes five or more tries for a kid to eat a new food. Be patient and keep trying. After a few tries, believe them when they say they don't like something and replace it with something else. We all dislike some foods.

Fruit is a part of every dinner at our house, every day, and the kids do eat it. Again, don't mention that it is good for you. Especially for the younger ones, encourage them by focusing on the good taste. Say something like, "Mmm, isn't this peach so sweet? I bet it was just picked from the peach tree yesterday, and the farmer had to fight the birds away because they wanted it!"

Don't be the parent who believes that kids won't eat their fruit. Of course they enjoy fruit. But be realistic. Depending on their age, they may not eat that whole piece of fruit that you put in their lunches. And if you give them an apple in their lunch when they expect a cookie, don't think that they will actually eat the apple. Our generation has not solved this old dilemma, and no generation ever will. As long as some school kids have junk food in their lunches, then whole pieces of fruit are doomed.

How many adults do you know who will eat an apple or banana right after they've had their sandwich at lunchtime? Very few. Who even thinks about adding fruit to their lunches? The only time I've seen adults eat a whole piece of fruit is at the pick-your-own fruit farms. It is actually quite fun watching adults sneaking free apples and peaches in these orchards. Your best offense is to include fruits at breakfast and dinner.

My husband gets credit for creating a fruit stand in our kitchen when our kids were young. The fruit stand was table level so the kids could help themselves. And they did! I would find banana peels and fruit pits at their play desks. Young kids love feeling they are getting away with something when they can eat when they want to.

Best yet, my daughters did not know what soft drinks were until they were about six or seven. Even then, they didn't drink them except at birthday parties where I had no control. My secret was to tell them that kids thought they tasted bitter, and it worked. I cringe every time I see a parent let their young ones drink that stuff. More nutritious milk and fruit juices are available everywhere, even at fast-food places, and they always have been.

My motto was simple: it was my fault if my young kids ate junk food. No excuses. Be a strong parent, not their best friend. If you find yourself starting to cave, picture what your adult children will tell you about what they would have wanted while they were growing up. Your good judgment, coupled with common sense and lots of love, is all you need. Not food love, but good old hugs-and-kisses love. Don't be a parenting fool and console with food. Except with that occasional piece of outrageous chocolate cake!

38

Join the Food Revolution

I feel violated by unscrupulous food industry members and food marketers that have taken advantage of me. I especially feel violated because there is no powerful, moral watchdog to protect me from them. I am on my own. We have all read the numerous books on the lack of food safety, horrendous animal abuses, and dangerous chemicals, including pesticides and hormones. We also know there is a lack of government oversight, with some industries left to monitor themselves. We have all watched the documentaries. I have been manipulated and fooled by packaging, serving sizes, mislabeled organic food (when in fact they are not), misleading health benefits, over-processed foods with disguised ingredients, foods from foreign countries that are not thoroughly inspected, and thousands of marketing gimmicks.

I also feel my personal space has been violated because we are inundated with nonstop health information from every source possible at every minute of the day. Everyone seems to be an expert, and everyone needs a platform to preach from. We are being bombarded from every direction to save ourselves from cancer, heart disease, even death. And worst of all, we are expected to digest and analyze this information and use all of it in our daily lives.

Yet no one concurs on the specifics. No one tells us who the liars are. One moment our focus is sugar, then it's salt, then it's butter. The next moment it's oils, meats, eggs, hormones and antibiotics in milk and meats. We're told to be wary of produce from other countries, genetically engineered foods, substitute sugars, and soft drinks. We are also told to look closely at farm-raised seafood, canned foods and pre-packaged foods. Even the way we cook foods and the water we drink has been labeled harmful. Is there anything left?

For each and every item previously mentioned, there are health and science experts who can refute it. We can't even get experts to agree on the basics. You could spend a lifetime researching each food item without ever knowing if you have stumbled upon the truth. There is too much information, much of it contradictory. There are too many theories that, once benchmarks of the truth, are now either false or questionable. The food pyramid that generations used as a reference is now practically upside down. There is too much truthful information that manufacturers and marketers will vehemently refute because of profits. I am left to use my own judgment, and I want to strangle someone because my head is going to explode from this information overload.

So I am joining the food revolution that is gaining momentum throughout the nation. I am going back to basics and listening to Mother Nature. I will try to eat nature's bounty, just as most animals do, in its natural state whenever possible. I will eat moderately, just like animals. I will protect myself (as best I can) by including many food types so that I am covering all the bases for all my body parts. Gee, it almost sounds like good old common sense.

My Food Revolution

1. I will use my giant soup pot to make more homemade soups, stews, and main dishes to control fats, salt, and preservatives. This will also bring back the old-fashioned comfort food aspect that we all love.
2. I will eat basic foods in their natural state: fresh fruit, nuts, and vegetables. I will not overcook, over-salt, over-sugar, or over-butter.
3. I will start replacing canned, boxed, or over-processed food as best I can with foods in their natural state.
4. I will pay more attention to food labels.
5. I will proceed at a sensible pace so that I don't give up, saying to hell with it all.
6. I will include our beloved dog Ginger Rose in this revolution.

Conclusion

$\mathcal{L}$et's begin our journey and laugh our way to success!

We can be successful in our weight loss goals, ultimately becoming healthier, happier, and less stressed. All we need to do is take a new, more optimistic approach to diet and exercise. Let's start by eliminating from our lives all the diet and exercise bullshit containing negativity and unrealistic requirements. We don't need starvation diets or punishing workouts to improve our body and mind. We don't need self-help gurus telling us to love ourselves or zealous preachers pretending to know the word of God and promising that he will miraculously make us all thin if we just pray. And we certainly don't need celebrities who receive endorsement checks for participating in weight-loss plans reminding us that we have to do all the work ourselves—including paying for packaged foods and guidance. We especially don't need skinny people yelling obscenities at us and calling us losers because we won't adopt their restrictive eating style. We don't need gimmicks or promises of miracles. Let's banish this bullshit once and for all.

Instead, let's tell it like it is regarding why you overeat and why you have failed to lose the weight. Then follow a simple five-step plan to guide us to our weight-loss goals. Let's incorporate our personal strengths and knowledge gained through life experiences and good old common sense.

Tell all diet gurus, fitness experts, and skinny people to go to hell. Free your mind and spirit from all the diet and exercise BS that has led to desperation and failure. Begin a new, positive direction by replacing the words *diet* and *exercise*. Try *big kitako removal* instead of *diet* to keep your common sense about eating and *free spirit time* for *exercise* to set the tone for positive workout experiences. Instead of stressing over weight loss, laugh your way through it. No more obsessing or negative, destructive emotional battles. Positive energy will make the journey easier and more pleasant.

Go ahead, choose those new humorous, inspirational words to replace *diet* and *exercise* and laugh your way to becoming healthier. Future conversations with friends and family regarding weight will be about how hilarious your new words for *diet* and *exercise* are, how much calmer you feel since destroying the vile words, or about how you are finally kicking the devil's butt!

Start making those small changes that will lead to magnificent permanent results. One change we can make is to stop behaviors based on tradition that may be detrimental to us, such as New Year's diet resolutions. Let's end this practice of using the first of the year to start our annual diet resolutions that we know we won't keep. Let's make New Year's Day Freedom From Dieting Day.

Completely change the focus of New Year's Day to a celebration of the new changes you have made to your life. Celebrate the New Year by proclaiming that you now eat a great breakfast every day and have outrageous poop, you now incorporate 10 new fruits and vegetables in your menus, or your new diet plan is the "Kick Ass Plan." Every small change that becomes permanent is a reason to *celebrate* us every January 1st.

Let's have fun with our new Big Kitako Removal Plan by assigning the four-pig restaurant rating system to our local restaurants to remind us how to make healthier food and drink choices. It will also remind us that the location, atmosphere, and company are just as important, or even more important, than the food.

Declare victory that we are no longer diet fools, because we now know how to count calories, cook more creatively, and guide our kids. Sing "Hallelujah!" that our must-have junk foods can be a part of our plan—especially chocolate, which is a wonderful gift from nature.

Let's help our planet and ourselves by joining the Food Revolution. Respect nature and what it has to offer us. Keep foods in their natural state whenever possible, free of over-processing through added fats, sugars, hormones, and manmade preservatives. Enjoy the earth's bounty and make small steps toward becoming a vegevore: give fruits, vegetables, and whole grains a more important role in your menus and decrease the importance of animal products.

Celebrate each small step that results in success. Rejoice as you gain more confidence and control. We may never lose all of those last pounds, but with determination we can lose weight using these strategies and become healthier. Even if we incorporate only a few simple lifestyle changes, we will significantly change our lives. Let's give it a try.

Imagine people all over the world reexamining what *diet* and *exercise* mean to them. Visualize the power they will gain by destroying these words and replacing them with positive, energizing words. Now imagine these same people choosing new words for diet and exercise in every language.

Let a new personal journey begin. If each of us incorporates just a few of these changes, after one year the results would be tremendous!

So join me in finally losing the last damn 10 pounds or 15, 20, 25....

12-Month Plan

For those who would like a specific, more detailed plan to follow, I have outlined a 12-month, step-by-step guide.

Each month-long discussion on a specific topic will give us a better understanding of it and give us time for trial and error. Permanent change takes time, and each of us will find our "Aha!" moments at different stages. This is not a one-size-fits-all plan. The purpose of this book is for you to discover what works for you, just as I did. For example, choosing a new word for *diet* may come easily for some, but others may take longer to erase *diet* from their vocabulary.

Incorporate as many of these lifestyle changes as you can, and significantly change your life.

Month

1   Stop being a diet fool: Learn all about current and past diet gimmicks and stop throwing money at them (see chapter 13).

2   "Aha!" moment: Learn the truth about overeating (see chapter 2).

3   Obliterate words: Create new words for diet and exercise (see chapters 16 and 22).

4   Declare your life joys: Food will no longer be your priority (see chapter 18).

5   Become a vegevore: Add more fruits, vegetables, and whole grains to your menus (see chapter 24).

6   Let's talk about poop: Add more fiber to your menus (see chapter 27).

7   Learn food basics: Discover why certain foods are good for you (see chapter 23).

8   Baby steps: Small changes will give you significant results (see chapters 19 and 20).

9   Go green: Add calmness to your life (see chapter 21).

10   Learn to count calories: Change your portion sizes (see chapter 26).

11   Food revolution: Change the way you cook and view recipes (see chapter 38).

12   Bad to the bone: Learn about food cravings (see chapter 31).

References

"6 Small Meals vs. 3 Squares: Which is Better?" Women's Health America. Accessed March 3, 2011. http://womenshealth.com/component/content/article/47-womens-health-acess/591-6-small.

Agency for Toxic Substances and Disease Registry. *ToxFAQs for Tri-chloroethylene (TCE) (Tricloroetileno)*. Atlanta: Agency for Toxic Substances and Disease Registry, July 2003. http://www.atsdr.cdc.gov/toxfaqs/tf.asp?id=172&tid=30.

"Almonds nutrition facts." www.nutrition-and-you.com. Accessed March 3, 2011. http://www.nutrition-and-you.com/almonds.html.

"Alphabetical list of vegetables." Chris and Nic's Recipes. Accessed March 3, 2011. http://cookery.newarchaeology.com/vegetables.php.

"A-Z list of fruits." Chris and Nic's Recipes. Accessed March 3, 2011. http://cookery.newarchaeology.com/fruits.php.

Campbell, T. Collin, and Thomas M. Campbell II. *The China Study: The Most Comprehensive Study of Nutrition Ever Conducted and the Startling Implications for Diet, Weight Loss, and Long-term Health.* Dallas, TX: BenBella Books, 2006.

ChooseMyPlate.gov. US Department of Agriculture. Accessed June 1, 2011. http://www.choosemyplate.gov.

"Coconut: The Tree of Life." Coconut Research Center. 2004. http://www.coconutresearchcenter.org/.

"Does this menopause make me look fat?" BodyLogicMD. Accessed February 28, 2011. http://www.bodylogicmd.com/for-women/hormones-and-weight-gain.

Donner, Ed. "Why Men Burn Calories Faster." LIVESTRONG.COM. Last updated January 19, 2011. http://www.livestrong.com/article/360810-why-men-burn-calories-faster/.

Duffy, Linda. "Overweight doctors, nurses and the US Surgeon General." Examiner. July 25, 2009. http://www.examiner.com/low-carb-in-denver/overweight-doctors-nurses-and-the-us-surgeon-general.

"Food Cravings." RealLifeFood.com. Accessed February 28, 2011. http://www.reallifefood.com/Cravings.html.

Guimond, Laura. "'Vegevores' Swarm Oregon Convention Center." *Portland Spoke*. September 1, 2010. http://www.portlandspoke.com/2010/09/01/vegevores-swarm-oregon-convention-center/.

Hatfield, Heather. "The Scoop on Poop." WebMD. Accessed March 3, 2011. http://women.webmd.com/pharmacist-drugs-medication-9/digestive-problems.

"House plants as a living air purifier." Home-Air-Guide.com. Accessed March 3, 2011. http://www.home-air-guide.com/living-air-purifier.html.

Hume, Ed. "Houseplants That Help Purify The Air." Ed Hume Seeds. Accessed March 3, 2011. http://humeseeds.com/purify.htm.

Magee, Elaine. "Managing Menopause Symptoms Through Diet." MedicineNet.com. Accessed March 3, 2011. http://www .medicinenet.com/script/main/art.asp?articlekey=59895.

Mayo Clinic staff. "Counting calories: Get back to weight-loss basics." Mayo Clinic. December 19, 2009. http://www.mayoclinic.com/ health/calories/WT00011.

Moriyama, Naomi, and William Doyle. *Japanese Women Don't Get Old or Fat: Secrets of My Mother's Tokyo Kitchen.* New York, NY: Random House, 2005.

Mulrooney, Marie. "How Many Calories Are Burned During a 40 Min. Brisk Walk?" LIVESTRONG.COM. Last updated November 10, 2010. http://www.livestrong.com/article/303605-how-many-calories-are-burned-during-a-40-min.

Occupational Safety and Health Administration. "Benzene." US Department of Labor. Accessed March 3, 2011. http://www.osha .gov/SLTC/benzene.

Occupational Safety and Health Administration. "Formaldehyde." US Department of Labor. Accessed March 3, 2011. http://www .osha.gov/SLTC/formaldehyde.

Osterweil, Neil. "Fighting 40s Flab." MedicineNet.com. Last editorial review October 19, 2004. http://www.medicinenet.com/script/ main/art.sp?articlekey=56912.

Reuters Health, "Study Sheds Light on Sweet and Salty Cravings." PreventDisease .com. Accessed March 3, 2011. http://preventdisease.com/news/ articles/sweet_or_salty.shtml.

"Small meals and cholesterol." Cleveland Clinic. Accessed March 3, 2011. http://my.clevelandclinic.org/heart/prevention/askdietician/ask4_02.aspx.

USDA National Nutrient Database for Standard Reference, Release 23. Accessed March 3, 2011. http://www.ars.usda.gov/ba/bhnrc/ndl.

US Department of Agriculture and US Department of Health and Human Services. *Dietary Guidelines for Americans, 2010.* 7th edition. Washington, DC: US Government Printing Office, December 2010. http://www.health.gov/dietaryguidelines/ dga2010/DietaryGuidelines2010.pdf.

Vorvick, Linda J. "Fiber." MedlinePlus. Last updated February 28, 2011. http://www.nlm.nih.gov/medlineplus/ency/article/002470.htm.

"What are 'discretionary calories'?" US Department of Agriculture. Last updated February 9, 2011. http://www.mypyramid.gov/pyramid/discretionary_calories.html.

Winfrey, Oprah. "How Did I Let This Happen Again?" *O, The Oprah Magazine,* January 2009. http://www.oprah.com/spirit/Oprahs-Battle-with-Weight-Gain-O-January-2009-Cover/1.